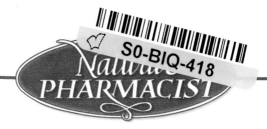

S0-BIQ-418

Nature's
PHARMACIST

Inside—Find the Answers to These Questions and More

☑ Can gingko delay the decline in memory of someone who has Alzheimer's disease? (See page 39.)

☑ What about in people with normal age-related memory loss? (See page 49.)

☑ How does it work? (See page 8.)

☑ What form of ginkgo is best to take, and how much should I use? (See page 55.)

☑ How long do I have to take it before I start seeing results? (See page 61.)

☑ Are there any side effects I should know about? (See page 69.)

☑ Are there any drugs that should not be combined with ginkgo? (See page 63.)

☑ Can L acetylcarnitine slow the progression of Alzheimer's disease? (See page 99.)

☑ I've heard the buzz about phosphatidylserine; what are the facts? (See page 91.)

☑ What two treatments for memory loss are sold as supplements but are more like drugs? (See pages 102 and 105.)

THE NATURAL PHARMACIST Library

Arthritis

Diabetes

Echinacea and Immunity

Feverfew and Migraines

Garlic and Cholesterol

Ginkgo and Memory

Heart Disease Prevention

Herbs

Illnesses and Their Natural Remedies

Kava and Anxiety

Menopause

PMS

Reducing Cancer Risk

Saw Palmetto and the Prostate

St. John's Wort and Depression

Vitamins and Supplements

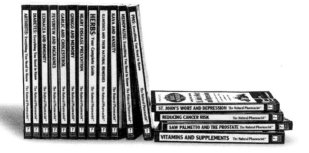

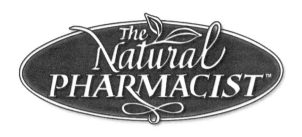

Everything You Need to Know About

Ginkgo
and Memory

Steven Dentali, Ph.D.

Series Editors

Steven Bratman, M.D.

David Kroll, Ph.D.

A DIVISION OF PRIMA PUBLISHING

Visit us online at www.thenaturalpharmacist.com

Warning—Disclaimer

This book is not intended to provide medical advice and is sold with the understanding that the publisher and the author are not liable for the misconception or misuse of information provided. The author and Prima Publishing shall have neither liability nor responsibility to any person or entity with respect to any loss, damage, or injury caused or alleged to be caused directly or indirectly by the information contained in this book or the use of any products mentioned. Readers should not use any of the products discussed in this book without the advice of a medical professional.

The Food and Drug Administration has not approved the use of any of the natural treatments discussed in this book. This book, and the information contained herein, has not been approved by the Food and Drug Administration.

Pseudonyms are used throughout to protect the privacy of the individuals involved.

PRIMA HEALTH and colophon are trademarks of Prima Communications, Inc.

THE NATURAL PHARMACIST™ is a trademark of Prima Communications, Inc.

All products mentioned in this book are trademarks of their respective companies.

Library of Congress Cataloging-in-Publication Data

Dentali, Steven.
    Ginkgo and memory / Steven Dentali.
      p. cm.—(The natural pharmacist)
    Includes bibliographical references and index.
    ISBN 0-7615-1552-6
    1. Ginkgo—Therapeutic use.   2. Alzheimer's disease—Alternative treatment.
3. Nootropic agents.   4. Memory.   I. Title.   II. Series.
RM666.G489D46   1998
616.8'0461—dc21   98-50708
                                           CIP

00 01 02 HH 10 9 8 7 6 5 4 3
Printed in the United States of America

Visit us online at www.thenaturalpharmacist.com

Contents

What Makes This Book Different?

The interest in natural medicine has never been greater. According to the National Association of Chain Drug Stores, 65 million Americans are using natural supplements, and the number is growing! Yet, it is hard for the consumer to find trustworthy sources for balanced information about this emerging field. Why? Frankly, natural medicine has had a checkered history. From snake oil potions sold at the turn of the century to those books, magazines, and product catalogs that hype miracle cures today, this is a field where exaggerated claims have been the norm.

Proponents of natural medicine have tended to abuse science, treating it more as a marketing tool than a means of discovering the truth.

But there is truth to be found. Studies of vitamins, minerals, and other food supplements have been with us since these nutritional substances were first discovered, and the level and quality of this science has grown dramatically in the last 20 years. Herbal medicine has been neglected in the United States, but in Europe, this, the oldest of all healing arts, has been the subject of tremendous and ongoing scientific interest.

At present, for a number of herbs and supplements, it is possible to give reasonably scientific answers to the questions: How well does this work? How safe is it? What types of conditions is it best used for?

THE NATURAL PHARMACIST series is designed to cut through the hype and tell you what we know and what we don't know about popular natural treatments. These books are more conservative than any others available, more honest about the weaknesses of natural approaches, more fair in their comparisons of natural and conventional treatments. You won't find any miracle cures here, but you will discover useful options that can help you become healthier.

Why Choose Natural Treatments?

Although the science behind natural medicine continues to grow, this is still a much less scientifically validated field than conventional medicine. You might ask, "Why should I resort to an herb that is only partly proven, when I could take a drug with solid science behind it?" There are at least three good reasons to consider natural alternatives.

First, some herbs and supplements offer benefits that are not matched by any conventional drug. Vitamin E is a good example. It appears to help prevent prostate cancer, a benefit that no standard medication can claim. Also, vitamin E almost certainly helps prevent heart disease. While there are standard drugs that also prevent heart disease, vitamin E works differently and may be able to complement many of the other approaches.

Another example is the herb milk thistle. Studies strongly suggest that this herb can protect the liver from injury. There is no pill or tablet your doctor can prescribe to do the same.

Even if the science behind some of these treatments is less than perfect, when the risks are low and the possible benefit high, a natural treatment may be worth trying. It is a little-known fact that for many conventional treatments the science is less than perfect as well, and physicians must balance uncertain benefits against incompletely understood risks.

A second reason to consider natural therapies is that some may offer benefits comparable to those of drugs with fewer side effects. The herb St. John's wort is a good example. Reasonably strong scientific evidence suggests that this herb is an effective treatment for mild to moderate depression, while producing fewer side effects on average than conventional medications. Saw palmetto for benign enlargement of the prostate, ginkgo for relieving symptoms and perhaps slowing the progression of Alzheimer's disease, and glucosamine for osteoarthritis are other examples. This is not to say that herbs and supplements are completely harmless—they're not—but for most the level of risk is quite low.

Finally, there is a philosophical point to consider. For many people, it "feels" better to use a treatment that comes from nature instead of from a laboratory. Just as you might rather wear all-cotton clothing than polyester, or look at a mountain landscape rather than the skyscrapers of a downtown city, natural treatments may simply feel more compatible with your view of life. We can quibble endlessly about just what "natural" means and whether a certain treatment is "actually" natural or not, but such arguments are beside the point. The difference is in the feeling, and feelings matter. In fact, having a good feeling about taking an herb may lead you to use it more consistently than you would a prescription drug.

Of course, at times synthetic drugs may be necessary and even lifesaving. But on many other occasions it may be quite reasonable to turn to an herb or supplement instead of a drug.

To make good decisions you need good information. Unfortunately, while hundreds of books on alternative medicine are published every year, many are highly misleading. The phrase "studies prove" is often used when the studies in question are so small or so badly conducted that they prove nothing at all. You may even find that the "data" from other books comes from studies with petri dishes and not real people!

You can't even assume that books written by well-known authors are scientifically sound. Many of these authors rely on secondary writers, leading to a game of "telephone," where misconceptions are passed around from book to book. And there's a strong tendency to exaggerate the power of natural remedies, whitewashing them with selective reporting.

THE NATURAL PHARMACIST series gives you the balanced information you need to make informed decisions about your health needs. Setting a new, high standard of accuracy and objectivity, these books take a realistic look at the herbs and supplements you read about in the news. You will encounter both favorable and unfavorable studies in these pages and will learn about both the benefits and the risks of natural treatments.

THE NATURAL PHARMACIST series is the source you can trust.

Steven Bratman, M.D.
David Kroll, Ph.D.

Introduction

Life in the "information age" can be hard on our memory. Each day it seems that the pace of life speeds up, with technology bringing us more and more information even as we seem to have less time in which to absorb it. In the modern world, we often find ourselves puzzling to remember a name or appointment, or leaving the grocery store wondering what important item we've forgotten to buy *this* time.

People of all ages have occasional slips of memory, but we tend to experience more of them as we get older. In fact, a gradual decline in memory is a natural part of growing old. Our brains' system for storing and retrieving memories loses some of its capacity as we age. If you think of memory as a physical function that depends on a good blood supply and adequate levels of key chemicals, it makes sense that old age (and stress) can impair memory somewhat.

Mild memory loss due to age or stress is upsetting enough, even though it's entirely normal. But sometimes memory loss is a symptom of a truly serious condition—dementia. Dementia, a severe loss of memory and mental functions, can be caused by malnutrition, metabolic imbalances, prescription drugs, trauma, or brain tumors—and in many cases can be successfully treated or even reversed. But the most common causes of dementia are Alzheimer's disease, a progressive condition with no known cure, and brain damage due to strokes. The available medications may, at best, temporarily reduce the symptoms or slow the advance of dementia.

A popular European herbal remedy may offer another option. The ginkgo tree, one of the oldest trees on earth, provides an herbal treatment that has been shown to help people suffering from dementia caused by Alzheimer's disease and other age-related conditions. Ginkgo seems to work about as well as prescription drugs used to treat dementia, and with fewer side effects. But keep in mind that only a proper medical evaluation can tell you whether the memory loss is a sign of a serious condition. Make sure to have a full medical evaluation before self-treating with ginkgo.

Ginkgo is also widely used by healthy people for ordinary memory loss. While there has been little scientific study of this use of ginkgo, there are logical reasons to believe that it might work. Research indicates that ginkgo is effective for different types of dementia arising from different causes. This suggests that ginkgo may be generally helpful for the brain's memory functions regardless of cause.

In this book we will examine the evidence for ginkgo, its safety, how to take it, what precautions to keep in mind, and what results to expect. We'll also introduce you to other natural substances used to improve memory and mental function, such as phosphatidylserine, L-acetylcarnitine, and ginseng. Then we'll objectively weigh the pros and cons of the drugs now used to treat dementia. Finally, we will address simple techniques and practices that can improve your ability to remember.

When you've read this book, you'll be acquainted with practically all the options to improve memory and mental function for yourself and your loved ones.

What Is Ginkgo?

Ginkgo has become a "hot" topic. From television programs to magazine articles and from teas and tinctures to a host of ginkgo-related products, this herb has been getting a lot of attention. According to a recent report, ginkgo was one of the top-selling herbs in the United States throughout 1997.[1]

Is ginkgo something you need to know about? Perhaps you have been wondering what it does, what it can do for you, and whether it is safe to use as a supplement. This book should be able to answer all your questions. We'll start with a description of the plant itself.

The Ginkgo Tree

The natural product extract that is receiving all this attention comes from the ginkgo, or maidenhair, tree. This unique tree, known scientifically as *Ginkgo biloba* L.,[2] is considered a "living fossil" because it existed at least 230 million years ago, in the early Paleozoic era.[3] Dinosaurs probably snacked on the same tree you can find along the streets of major cities today. There aren't many plants or animals from that era that still survive today.

Fossils of ginkgo's fan-shaped leaves date back at least 230 million years.

Ginkgo is the sole survivor of a prehistoric family of trees that thrived in Europe until the last ice age, when the ginkgo family was completely wiped out as huge sheets of ice swept across the continent. The ginkgo tree survived in China[4] and was later cultivated by Chinese monks.[5]

The ginkgo tree is extremely hardy, and individual trees can be very long-lived. Some have been known to survive for more than 1,000 years. One estimate even puts the life span of an individual ginkgo at 2,000 to 4,000 years![6]

Why Is It Called Ginkgo?

The name *ginkgo* comes from the nut (technically called the "ovule") produced by the female ginkgo tree. This primitive yellow-green seed ripens to an orange-brown, foul-smelling, and fleshy "fruit" that encloses a silvery inner kernel. This kernel is what actually gives ginkgo its common name. The term comes from the Japanese word *ginkyo: gin* meaning silver, and *kyó* meaning apricot. This "silver apricot" has been specially prepared, usually by boiling or roasting, and eaten in the Orient for thousands of years.

The species name, *biloba,* comes from the tree's un-usual leaves. The fan-shaped leaves of ginkgo have an in-dentation or a split down the middle. Because of this split, botanists consider it two-lobed, or *bilobed.*

Arising from the Ashes

The legendary hardiness and survivability of the ginkgo tree was demonstrated in Hiroshima, Japan, in the '40s. A ginkgo tree located in the city center was incinerated along with all other plants and animals when the atomic bomb detonated on August 6, 1945. The following year, a new ginkgo tree sprouted where the old one had been and grew into a normal, full-sized tree.[7]

What Does the Ginkgo Look Like?

Although you might not have been aware of it, you've probably already seen a ginkgo tree. Because this specimen is so hardy that it's very tolerant of pollution and resistant to insect attack, ginkgo is popular with urban planners. Consequently, these trees can be found in many large cities throughout Europe and North America.

Like most trees, the ginkgo is easiest to identify by its leaves (see figure 1). The distinctive, fan-shaped leaf can grow to a size large enough to just about cover the palm of your hand. The leaf fan extends from a stalk that comes directly from the stem of the tree. As mentioned earlier, the leaf fan usually has a split or indention in the middle, creating the two-lobed effect for which the tree was named. Note that the smaller and younger leaves of the ginkgo tree may not be split and that older ones may have more than a single indentation.

If you compare a ginkgo leaf to the leaves of other trees, you'll certainly notice the difference. Ginkgo leaves lack the fine cross-vein structure of other leaves and instead have veins that radiate or "fan" out from the base of the leaf to its edges. The effect is much like that of a Chinese fan.

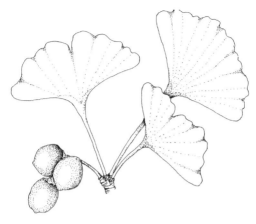

Figure 1. *Leaves of the ginkgo tree*

The ginkgo tree is *deciduous,* which means that it sheds its leaves in the fall, like many other trees do. Green in the summer, the ginkgo's leaves turn a glowing yellow in the autumn.

Ginkgos can grow to 130 feet in height. Trees that haven't yet reached maturity are shaped like a cone. Without their leaves, younger branches look like they've been fashioned from coat hangers, as they split off the main trunk at almost right angles. As ginkgo trees get older and larger, they develop more of a spreading crown. The ginkgo tree is so distinctive that once you've identified your first ginkgo, you'll likely be able to identify others even after they've lost their leaves.

What Is in Ginkgo?

Green plants are virtual chemical factories, and the ginkgo tree is no exception. The ginkgo spends its days absorbing sunlight, water, and nutrients from the soil and producing chemicals that help it grow. Two types of chemicals produced by the ginkgo tree are of particular interest to us: *flavonoids* and *terpenes.*

Flavonoids are common in our everyday lives. In fact, if you eat 3 to 5 servings of fruits and vegetables daily, then you're probably consuming a gram of these substances a day, which can be beneficial to your health. Many flavonoids have an antioxidant effect similar to that of vitamins E and C.

You've probably seen a ginkgo tree; they're found in many cities.

Flavonoids, which are found in all flowering plants, are the chemicals that give leaves their fall colors. Most of the flavonoids found in ginkgo are commonly found in many other plants.

Terpenes, another class of chemicals found in plants, are substances that help produce a plant's characteristic odor. The scent of a rose or the fragrance of an orange blossom are both the result of evaporating terpenes. Ginkgo produces certain unique terpenes, called *ginkgolides* and *bilobilade.* Although many other chemical substances are found in ginkgo, modern research into the plant's medicinal properties has concentrated mostly on flavonoids and terpenes.

What Was Ginkgo Used for Historically?

The medicinal use of ginkgo goes back about 5,000 years to the beginning of traditional Chinese medicine. In the *Pen Ts'ao Ching,* China's first-known classic herbal book, ginkgo seeds and fruit were recommended for treating conditions involving the heart and lungs. In the 1700s, ginkgo was brought to Europe as an ornamental tree, but the European herbalists of the time did not use it. Not until this century did ginkgo become of interest to the

The European Versus U.S. View of Herbs

The different attitudes toward ginkgo in the United States and Europe reflect how the different cultures regard herbal medicines. Over the years, both the physicians and pharmaceutical companies of Europe have maintained an active interest in herbal treatments.

European researchers have asked two basic questions about these natural remedies:

- Do they really work?
- How do we know how well they can work compared to conventional medications?

Western world. This time, medical scientists focused on the leaf instead of the fruit.

Entry into Modern Medicine

During the 1930s, European interest in the medicinal properties of flavonoids drew researchers' attention to the ginkgo leaf as a particularly rich source of these chemicals.[8] A concentrated extract of these flavonoids became the basis for study. In 1965, this ginkgo extract was registered for use in Germany.[9] The French medical journal *La Presse Médicale* devoted its entire September 25 issue to studies of an extract of this remarkable plant.

What Is Ginkgo Used for Today?

In Europe today, ginkgo is primarily used for treating age-related memory loss. In Germany, it is among the top-

In many cases, modern scientific studies have provided ample evidence that herbal medications do indeed produce results. Many such products have been approved for use and incorporated into modern European medical care.

It's a different story here across the Atlantic. The once-burgeoning medicinal plant industry that supplied most of our medicines around the turn of the century is gone, and the experts of that time have disappeared along with it. For most of this century, herbal medicines have been considered "folk remedies." However, in the last few decades, attitudes appear to be changing. We are now seeing a renewed interest in both natural products and natural health care.

selling herb products prescribed by physicians. It is also among the most prescribed herbal remedies in France and is widely used in other European countries as well.

In the late 1980s, Germany's Commission E (the official body in charge of validating herbal use) authorized ginkgo for two major purposes:

- Improving mental function in the elderly
- Promoting circulation

In North America, however, ginkgo has not yet been embraced by conventional medicine. However, the herb has become one of the most popular "dietary supplements" on the market.

Strong scientific evidence tells us that ginkgo can improve memory and mental function. Its capacity to do so makes it a *nootropic agent,* a treatment that improves brain function. At this time, only two nootropic drugs have been approved in the United States to treat Alzheimer's disease: Cognex (tacrine) and Aricept (donepezil). If you are interested in reading more about them right now, see chapter 10. In chapters 4 and 9, we'll discuss evidence that ginkgo and certain other natural herbs and supplements may also improve memory and other aspects of mental capacity.

Ginkgo is widely used in Germany and France.

Considerable evidence suggests that ginkgo increases blood circulation in various parts of the body. Until the 1980s, researchers assumed that its beneficial effects on memory were due to increased blood flow to the brain. Recent research, however, has changed that thinking. Today, research suggests that ginkgo's effect on memory and its effect on circulation are two distinct functions.

Ginkgo's positive effect on circulation has led to its use in relieving "intermittent claudication," the severe leg cramps caused by hardening of the arteries. The herb has also been used to treat other conditions in which poor circulation is involved, including impotence, strokes, and the "cold hand" condition known as Raynaud's syndrome. (Please note that combining ginkgo with any of the blood-thinning medications that your physician may prescribe for these conditions may not be safe.)

One study suggests that ginkgo may be helpful in premenstrual tension syndrome (PMS). It has been also recommended for a number of other conditions such as allergies, asthma, and macular degeneration of the eye, although little to no evidence supports these uses.

An article published in *Time* magazine on November 3, 1997, has done much to boost public awareness of

Ginkgo biloba. Time reported the results of a study published in the *Journal of the American Medical Association* (*JAMA*). Known as the Le Bars study for its main author, this research examined the use of a special ginkgo extract in treating Alzheimer's disease and age-related memory loss. This study was especially notable to the American medical community since it was performed at six medical centers across the United States, enrolling a total of more than 300 patients. The results led to considerable excitement among the conventional medical community about ginkgo's potential. Ginkgo is now well on its way toward being an accepted medical treatment in this country.

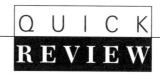

QUICK REVIEW

- *Ginkgo biloba* L., also known as the maidenhair tree, has been around since before the last ice age. The plant has no close relatives that exist today.

- Ginkgo contains chemicals called flavonoids and terpenes. The terpenes called *ginkgolides* and *bilobalide* are unique to ginkgo.

- The fruit and seeds of ginkgo have long been used in China as a treatment for a variety of conditions.

- In Europe, a special extract of ginkgo leaf has been an accepted medical treatment since at least the late 1980s. It is used for memory loss and mental decline in the elderly, as well as for decreased blood circulation. A recent study conducted in the United States has paved the way for increased acceptance of ginkgo in North America.

CHAPTER

T W O

Age-Related Memory Loss

W e all forget things. We leave the house without our car keys and forget the names that go with the faces we meet. We leave home without our shopping lists and forget phone numbers we once knew. And the older we get, the more frequently these episodes seem to occur. Whether this is happening to us or to a parent or loved one, our forgetfulness gives us cause for discomfort and reflection. Is this memory loss part of the normal process of aging? Or is it a warning sign of something more serious? And of course, we wonder, can we do anything about it?

The Good News and the Bad

If you're troubled because your memory is no longer what it once was, you may be relieved to know that what you are experiencing is probably a normal part of the aging process. Studies using sophisticated batteries of tests have shown that memory usually declines with advancing age, beginning at about age 40.

It is important to note that this condition, known as Age-Related Cognitive Decline (ARCD) or Age-Associated Memory Impairment (AAMI), is not a disease. Age-related memory loss is a natural part of growing older, and it happens to us all. What's the good news, you ask? The good news is that there *is* much that we can do to better cope with a slipping memory. Even more important, there may be steps we can take to slow or even stop this decline. This book will tell you what we know and what we still only guess in this rapidly evolving field.

What *Kind* of Memory Loss?

We go to the doctor when we are not feeling well. We go when we've noticed a physical change, be it a lump or a pain. We go for headaches, backaches, and blurred vision, but we seldom go for a bad memory. We naturally, and usually correctly, assume that growing slightly forgetful is simply a normal part of growing older. However, this is not always the case.

If you are experiencing memory loss, it is important to keep in mind that it might *not* mean *age-related* memory loss. There are other causes of memory impairment, many of which require early diagnosis as well as early treatment. These possibilities include problems with prescription medications, chemical imbalances, or the more dreaded possibilities of Alzheimer's disease, strokes, and brain tumors. Such health-threatening conditions or diseases need to be diagnosed and treated by a medical doctor.

In the next chapter, I discuss some of these more serious causes of memory loss. To be on the safe side, if you are experiencing memory loss, seeing your physician to first rule out a more serious condition is important. This visit to your doctor may be useful to get a "baseline" clinical evaluation of your cognitive functions. Then, if you have such tests performed again at intervals, your doctor can determine how quickly your memory might be failing and whether your forgetfulness is an indicator of a more serious condition. Based on this information, you can decide what steps you should take.

Ginkgo may be an effective way to combat memory loss of various types. If you wish to skip directly to the chapters that discuss ginkgo, turn to chapters 5 and 6 to learn how to take ginkgo and how you can use it safely and successfully.

How Our Memories Work

Have you ever wondered *how* you think and remember? While there has been extensive scientific investigation into this field, exactly how our memories function remains a mystery. Although we understand a great deal about the brain and nervous system, when it comes to how thoughts and memory are actually stored, there are enormous gaps in our knowledge.

Many causes of memory impairment require early diagnosis and treatment.

Thought and memory involve a complex network of microscopic nerve cells known as *neurons,* all connected to the "central clearinghouse," our brain. These nerve cells are connected end-to-end everywhere throughout our bodies, and information travels along this vast network of "wiring" through a combination of electrical current and a complex series of chemical interactions. The chemical interactions take place at the gaps between nerve endings, where one neuron ends and another begins. These important "intersections" are known as *synapses.*

When this network breaks down and nerve transmissions can no longer reach their intended destinations, mental functions fail. Certain chemicals play a critical role by enabling nerve signals to cross synapses. Among the most important of these chemical transmitters is *acetylcholine.* Without adequate levels of acetylcholine, memory and mental function are inevitably impaired. Certain drugs and natural treatments for memory loss are thought to work by augmenting the effects of acetylcholine.

Phospholipids are also important in helping nerve cells function properly. They don't affect neurotransmission; rather, phospholipids are vital components of cell membranes. These membranes affect nerve impulse conduction by controlling the gathering, storing, and release of neurotransmitters, and may help determine how

> **It's important to know that by keeping your mind active and establishing good habits, you can overcome the slow deterioration of memory that normally occurs with age.**

long a nerve cell will function before it becomes useless and is destroyed. One phospholipid, phosphatidylserine (also known as PS), is a natural substance used to treat memory loss and declining mental function. We will return to this substance in chapter 8.

Our Memory Circuits

Memory depends on these "neural networks." It appears that different areas in our brains store different types of information, including sights, sounds, and smells. Thoughts

Mae's Story

Mae is an example of someone who worried about her failing memory. She'd been an executive secretary for nearly 28 years and was only a few years from retirement. Lately, however, she had begun to notice how easily she was forgetting things. Work seemed busier, more stressful, and more of a struggle. Phone calls would interrupt her train of thought, and afterwards she'd have trouble remembering what she'd been doing just before the call came in. From phone numbers to office supplies, it seemed like little things were tripping her up. Lately, she'd even forgotten one of her grandchildren's birthdays. Occasionally, she'd go into the kitchen only to discover that she couldn't remember why.

Mae visited her doctor hoping to understand why her memory seemed to be failing her more and more. After ques-

and memories travel along neural pathways and across the "synaptic connections" to and from the various storage areas in our brain. These connections play a major role in memory formation. They are much like the telephone circuits that carry messages across networks of wires and through complex switching systems. Our nervous system is marvelously designed to get the right message to the right place.

Say you meet a person for the first time. Virtually every detail about her—what she looks like, what she's wearing, the sound of her voice—travels to the various centers in your brain, "connecting" across the gaps between nerve cells to form a unique pathway. If you never see her again, this connection will fade over time. However, if you should tioning her for some time, her doctor suggested Mae cut back on some of her duties at work and lessen her commitments on the home front. In brief, he recommended that she reduce the stress caused by her busy life. She did as her doctor suggested, and Mae was pleased to find that—though her memory still wasn't completely reliable—she could remember more things more easily than she could just a few months previously. She was experiencing an effect of aging, but by changing her lifestyle, she improved her ability to concentrate and recall.

Mae's memory problems are what would be expected with the natural course of aging. Remembering names and details, learning new information, and maintaining a high level of concentration are all subject to the toll of the aging process.

see her again, or even think about her, the connection will strengthen. The more this pathway is used, the more permanent the connection becomes and the more permanent the memory becomes. This contributes to the difference between what we know as our short-term and long-term memories, and it also explains the important role repetition plays in our thought processes.

The Symptoms of Age-Related Memory Loss

For most of us, certain aspects of memory begin to deteriorate with age. We begin to have trouble remembering names, or we find ourselves in a room with no recollection of how we got there or why we went there (a symptom sometimes jokingly referred to as "destinesia"). These annoying memory lapses are perfectly normal. They don't mean that you have or are going to get Alzheimer's disease! It's important to know that by keeping your mind active and establishing good habits, you can overcome the slow deterioration of memory that normally occurs with age.

The Causes of Age-Related Memory Loss

The reasons we suffer gradual memory impairment as we age are many and complex. Causes of age-related memory loss are both physical and "functional." In other words, memory loss can be a result of both physical factors and behavioral and environmental factors.

Physical Causes

During the normal course of aging, our brains and nervous systems undergo a series of physical changes. Nerve cells work less effectively and don't make new connections as easily. This can inhibit our ability to form memories. Some nerve cells may die or suffer damage. Certain memory connections can also become lost. Finally, the concentration of certain brain chemicals may also diminish, impairing the brain's function.

Other physical problems associated with age may contribute more indirectly to memory loss. For example:

- Diminished eyesight or hearing can give us false perceptions and memories.
- Chronic illness can impair attention, focus, and therefore memory.
- Confusion, fatigue, or drowsiness caused by prescription or over-the-counter medications can decrease our awareness and ability to remember.

Functional Causes

Still other problems with memory may relate to aspects of lifestyle that go along with age. Part of the reason children have such good memories (except for their chores or homework assignments) is that they have less on their minds than older people do. Did you ever consider that stress, for example, has a bad effect on memory? Think about how easy it is to forget something when you are frustrated and in a hurry. And the older you are, the more responsibilities you may have that wear you down. Influences that contribute to memory problems include the following:

- Overload of information
- Stress
- Frustration
- Being in a hurry
- Lack of sleep
- Depression
- Lack of stimulation
- Worry
- Grief
- Alcohol and drug misuse
- Poor diet

Dealing with Age-Related Memory Loss

What is most remarkable about age-related memory impairment is that so many of its causes are treatable or simply *changeable.* Getting enough sleep, eating properly, working with your doctor to make sure you are taking only the medications you truly need, even having your glasses checked can make a big difference. Regularly exercising your mind can make a big difference as well. People who engage in stimulating intellectual activity may be helping themselves to strengthen and maintain mental function.

There are many techniques you can use to avoid memory lapses. In chapter 11, I provide memory aids and techniques to make your memory more effective. You may also find ginkgo and other natural treatments that are described in later chapters helpful.

When the Worst Happens

Sometimes memory loss is more severe than a simple lapse. Perhaps you're dealing with a parent or loved one who is suffering from symptoms of mental decline that seem more profound than the forgetfulness caused by aging. Serious disease or disorder may be at work, and recognizing this fact is extremely important. The following story illustrates this point.

Some problems with memory may relate to the way you live your life as you age.

Tom's daughter had become very worried about him. She'd gone to visit and found him in his pajamas, sitting in the garage. "I can't remember why I came out here," he told her. He seemed confused. She'd noticed other warning signs, too. Lately, he appeared to be spending much more time just sitting and staring out the window. He no longer kept the kitchen neat and clean as he had always done, and the refrigerator seemed uncharacteristically empty. It was becoming clear that he was no longer taking care of himself in the way that he had been. He often seemed distracted and distant.

Tom was indeed suffering from something more serious than simply a gradual memory loss. The rather abrupt interruption of his normal lifestyle as well as the dramatic change in his personality left Tom's daughter with no doubt that her father needed help. When she took him to the doctor, the diagnosis confirmed her worst fears. Her father was suffering from early Alzheimer's symptoms.

You may even wonder whether your own symptoms of memory loss might be worse than you should expect. Chances are they are not, but if you have any concerns of this type, I strongly recommend a comprehensive medical evaluation. In the next chapter, we'll consider some of the more serious causes of memory decline.

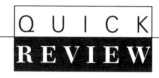

QUICK REVIEW

- A gradual decline in memory is a natural part of growing older.

- Our thoughts and memories are transmitted along the complex network that makes up our brain and nervous system. This system loses some of its capacity with age.

- Other possible factors contributing to age-related mental decline include fatigue, poor diet, failing eyesight, stress, and prescription medications.

- You can take steps to improve your memory, both by eliminating causes of poor memory and also by using memory-building techniques.

- In some cases, something more serious than ordinary age-related memory loss may be going on. If you are concerned that you or a loved one may be showing serious signs of declining mental function, make sure to have a full medical evaluation.

Could It Be Alzheimer's Disease?

F
ew things in life can bring us more heartbreak than watching a parent, spouse, or loved one sink into the abyss that is Alzheimer's disease. For family members and caregivers, this condition can bring feelings of hopelessness, helplessness, and pain.

This chapter presents the basic facts that we know about Alzheimer's disease—what it is, how to determine whether you or a loved one has it, and what to do about it. It also covers related diseases that may be mistaken for Alzheimer's.

Alzheimer's disease is the major cause of severe age-related memory loss and impaired mental function. Technically, this condition is called by the severe-sounding word "dementia." Dementia has several other possible causes in addition to Alzheimer's disease. Furthermore, other illnesses can present symptoms that on the surface resemble dementia, but are actually quite different. Because identifying precisely what disease you are dealing with can be crucial, this chapter briefly introduces the primary conditions that cause dementia.

What Is "Dementia"?

What we once knew as "senility," modern medicine now calls *dementia*. This term includes a variety of conditions, all of which are related to severe loss of memory and mental functions. These conditions are usually, though not always, associated with age. Alzheimer's disease is the cause of nearly 70% of all cases of true dementia.[1] The next most common cause of dementia is multiple small strokes, known as "multi-infarct dementia." There are other causes too, and we'll discuss some of them later in this chapter.

Alzheimer's disease is the cause of nearly 70% of all cases of true dementia.

People with dementia ultimately cannot care for themselves. Often, family members are the first to notice that something is wrong. And usually, these family members are also the ones who have to make arrangements to care for the relative as the disease progresses.

The case of 53-year-old Jennie is a typical example. One winter afternoon, she called her daughter and said that her jewelry box with more than $20,000 worth of jewels had disappeared. Naturally, her children were very concerned.

After an exhaustive search of the house, the jewelry box was found in the bottom of the freezer. This was only part of the surprise. Her family also found numerous other items she'd hidden around the house, including many packets of money. In all, they found nearly $10,000 in cash. Jennie had no recollection of hiding any of it.

Her family decided that this seemed more than just simple forgetfulness. Evaluations by both the family physician and a neurologist determined that she was suffering from early onset dementia, most likely from Alzheimer's disease.

The Importance of a Diagnosis

Keep in mind that memory loss and confusion do not always signal the onset of dementia due to Alzheimer's disease. Severe memory loss and mental impairment can result from any of a number of causes, many of which are treatable; some are even reversible. If the diagnosis *is* Alzheimer's disease, there are treatments as well. Although none can cure the disease, they can improve memory, mental function, and behavior for a while, and perhaps even slow the progression of the disease in some cases.

People with dementia ultimately cannot care for themselves.

These treatments include ginkgo, phosphatidylserine (also known as PS), L-acetylcarnitine, and approved conventional medications.

Many of the same treatments that help those who suffer from Alzheimer's disease can also be used for other forms of dementia, such as multi-infarct dementia. However, in some of these cases, simply taking a general treatment to improve memory and mental function would not make sense. More specific treatment might be much more effective.

The story of Susan is a good example. Retired and living at home with her husband of 30 years, Susan suddenly seemed to become confused and agitated. Her husband even found her walking around in the basement one morning. "I don't know why I came down here," she told him. She seemed distant, almost as if she were somewhere else.

His heart sank. Did she have Alzheimer's disease? But before jumping to conclusions, he took her to their family physician. The doctor looked at her chart, asked a few questions, and immediately suspected a sleeping medication she'd been taking. He switched her to a different medication, and within 2 days Susan was her old self again.

Proper medical diagnosis is a vital part of successful treatment.

Obviously, it would not have made sense to simply give Susan ginkgo! When there is an identifiable and treatable cause of mental impairment, it needs to be addressed. Later in the chapter, I will discuss some of the conditions that may masquerade as Alzheimer's disease. For now, the moral of the story is that proper medical diagnosis is a vital part of successful treatment.

Alzheimer's Disease

If you have a loved one who is suffering from Alzheimer's disease, learning as much about this disease process as you can is important. Understanding how the disease progresses will help you know what to expect and enable you to be more effective at dealing with it. Exploring every treatment possibility is also important, and ginkgo may be one of your options.

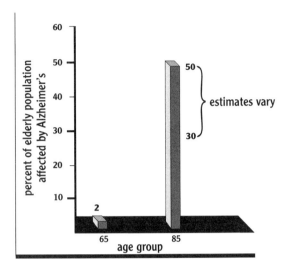

Figure 2. *Alzheimer's disease is rare in people younger than 65*

What Is Alzheimer's Disease?

While the effects of this disease are well known, what causes it and how it works are still something of a mystery. We do know that Alzheimer's disease affects brain tissue directly and that the result is a gradual destruction of brain cells. This is a disease that almost always affects people older than 65 years of age. Less than 2% of the elderly have Alzheimer's disease by the age of 65. That number increases to 30 to 50% by the age of 85 (see figure 2). While people younger than age 40 are sometimes affected, it is rare. At present, 4 million people in the United States alone are believed to be affected by this disease.[2]

The progression of Alzheimer's disease sometimes slows down or even stops for periods of time—occasionally for as long as several years. But eventually, the disease re-

The Alzheimer's Association

The Alzheimer's Association seeks to eliminate Alzheimer's disease through the advancement of research, while enhancing care and support services for individuals and their families. To locate the chapter nearest you, call 1-800-272-3900. The association has a home page on the World Wide Web of the Internet; the address is www.alz.org.

Another good site with great links for information on dementia and Alzheimer's disease is maintained by the Mayo Clinic. Their Internet address is www.mayohealth.org. This site is very informative, in fact one of the best I found on the subject. The National Institute of Mental Health also provides excellent information at www.nimh.nih.gov/publicat/alzheim.htm.

news its course. Alzheimer's disease usually results in death about 8 to 10 years after symptoms first appear. While Alzheimer's disease is not curable, it is treatable. This means that while nothing will stop this disease or reverse the damage that results, slowing the decline may be possible. Ginkgo may be one such treatment; the supplement phosphatidylserine appears to be another.

When to Suspect Alzheimer's Disease

Usually, people begin to suspect dementia due to Alzheimer's disease when symptoms of memory loss and mental impairment are more severe than would otherwise be expected. Where a person who is simply forgetful might not remember where his car keys are, someone with dementia from Alzheimer's disease might forget how to get to the market they've been going to for years. There are other important signs, too, and often a combination of them is what alarms the family. Here are a few:

Sudden disorientation to time and place. It is common in people suffering the onset of dementia from this disease to undergo a sudden disorientation to time or place. They might get "lost" at the mall or even in their own backyard. This can be a terrifying experience for both the victim and his or her loved ones.

Loss of judgment. Another signal of the onset of dementia due to Alzheimer's disease is loss of judgment. Martin, who had always managed his money carefully, is a good example of this. In his late 70s, Martin suddenly began to purchase numerous items over the television shopping channels. In the course of a few weeks, he had charged several thousand dollars worth of items, nearly all of which he had no use for.

Problems with abstract thinking. Everyday problems that require abstract thought can be difficult or even impossible for a person suffering from dementia due to Alzheimer's disease. Balancing the checkbook, recognizing numbers, and performing simple calculations may all seem to be as incomprehensible as a foreign language.

Misplacing things. We all misplace things from time to time, but a person with Alzheimer's disease is likely to put things in inappropriate places—such as Jennie putting her jewelry in the freezer—and have no memory of how they got there.

Other signs of dementia due to Alzheimer's disease include rapid changes in mood, sudden changes in personality, and a dramatic loss of initiative. This disease *seriously* disrupts a person's lifestyle. For example, your loved one may have been very active, whereas now she has suddenly become uninterested in her usual pursuits, wishing only to

The Alzheimer's Association
10 Warning Signs

- Memory loss that affects job skills
- Difficulty performing familiar tasks
- Problems with language
- Disorientation to time and place
- Poor or decreased judgment
- Problems with abstract thinking
- Misplacing things or putting them in inappropriate places
- Rapid changes in mood or behavior
- Changes in personality
- Loss of initiative and general noninterest in the usual pursuits

sit in front of the television all day. Or she may become suddenly suspicious or fearful of other people.

Making a Diagnosis of Alzheimer's Disease

Alzheimer's disease causes symptoms that fit into a general pattern; this pattern is what doctors look for. At present, we have no perfect technique for diagnosing Alzheimer's disease. No lab tests or x-ray measurements can make a definitive diagnosis. The only guaranteed way to identify Alzheimer's is to perform an autopsy of the brain! Doctors, therefore, must make their diagnosis by considering a patient's medical history, physical examinations, various tests of mental status, and (most important) by ruling out other possible diseases that might cause similar symptoms.

The Causes of Alzheimer's Disease

As mentioned earlier, more is known about what Alzheimer's disease does to the brain than what causes it. In fact, almost nothing is known for certain about the cause of this disease, except that nerve cells in the brain are damaged. Current theories include the suggestion that abnormal protein handling by the brain may play a role.[3] Other theories point to possible effects of substances such as aluminum[4] or zinc.[5]

Making the diagnosis of Alzheimer's disease includes ruling out other kinds of dementia.

It appears that levels of the brain chemical *acetylcholine* are affected by Alzheimer's disease. This important chemical, mentioned in chapter 2, is critical to the transmission of thought and memory. It appears that Alzheimer's disease gradually destroys nerve cells in the brain that produce acetylcholine.[6] Many of the treatments used for Alzheimer's disease are believed to work by boosting acetylcholine levels, perhaps enabling failing nerve cells to continue to function for a while (see chapter 10).

Other Kinds of Dementia

As we've mentioned earlier, Alzheimer's disease is not the only cause of dementia, only the most common.

Multi-Infarct Dementia

The second leading cause of dementia, after Alzheimer's disease, is *multi-infarct dementia.* It accounts for about 15% of dementia cases (see figure 3). Multi-infarct dementia results from a series of small "strokes" in the brain.

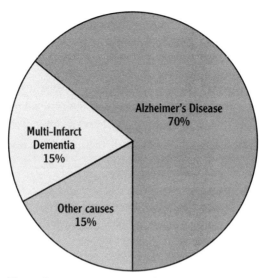

Figure 3. *Dementia is caused by various diseases*

Strokes occur when arteries in the brain become blocked, shutting off blood (and therefore oxygen) to areas of the brain "downstream." Such small strokes actually kill brain cells, and the affected area is known as an "infarct." These strokes are usually detectable by such tests as CT scans and MRI.

A small stroke in the areas of the brain involving thought processes and memory may impair mental functions slightly. When a series of such strokes occur, the symptoms of dementia become obvious.

The best approach to multi-infarct dementia is to treat the underlying causes and thereby prevent further small strokes. In most people, this means quitting smoking, improving diet, exercising, and taking other actions to lower blood pressure and cholesterol. (General advice on this subject may be found in *The Natural Pharmacist*

It Wasn't Alzheimer's Disease

The following story may sound unbelievable, but it happened. Richard was a nursing home resident with the diagnosis of dementia from Alzheimer's disease. He seldom got up from bed, didn't seem to recognize members of his family, and had trouble feeding himself. After a couple of years, however, a new physician took over the care of patients in the nursing home. Richard's new doctor found his case unusual. Over the many years Richard had been in the hospital, his condition had not gotten any worse. This didn't seem to fit with the diagnosis of Alzheimer's disease.

Guide to Heart Disease Prevention.) Treatments used for Alzheimer's disease may also help improve mental function in multi-infarct dementia.

Other Causes of Dementia

Other causes of dementia are more rare and include Parkinson's disease, AIDS, alcohol and drug abuse, Huntington's chorea, and multiple sclerosis. These forms of dementia can all produce symptoms similar to those caused by Alzheimer's disease. Since treatments vary for these forms of dementia, it is important that the specific cause be properly identified. Again, seeking the expertise of a doctor is crucial.

Diseases That Might Be Mistaken for Dementia

Most of us have heard the saying, "If it looks like a duck and quacks like a duck, it's a duck." When it comes to mental impairment in the elderly, however, it's easy to be fooled. Conditions that are not dementia at all are often

As an experiment, the physician gave Richard the antidepressant drug Zoloft. Within 4 weeks Richard was walking around and talking to the staff. A month later he went home, and soon he was driving again. He never had Alzheimer's disease; he had instead been suffering from a severe and chronic form of major depression.

The moral of the story is this: Don't assume symptoms of memory loss means Alzheimer's disease. Make sure you get a medical evaluation for yourself or your loved one!

—Steven Bratman, M.D.

mistaken for it, leading to inappropriate or delayed treatment. Finding out what is causing the symptoms of mental impairment is crucial for proper treatment of the problem.

Depression is the most common form of mental illness affecting the elderly, and it is mistaken for dementia so often that it has been called "pseudo-dementia." Even mild to moderate depression can produce a dementia-like memory loss. Sometimes, neither those suffering from significant depression nor their families recognize it as such. Again, proper medical diagnosis is very important. The really good news is that once depression is diagnosed, it is almost always treatable.

Other conditions that might produce the kinds of mental changes seen in dementia are brain tumors, malnutrition, metabolic imbalances, side effects of prescription medications, and trauma. Again, many of these causes are easily treated if identified.

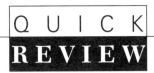

- Dementia, or what we used to know as "senility," causes severe loss of memory and mental functions.

- Proper medical diagnosis is an important step in treating any form of dementia. If you suspect that you or a loved one may be developing dementia from Alzheimer's disease, first see a doctor to rule out the possibility of another disease that might need specific treatment. Such conditions as depression, brain tumors, malnutrition, side effects from prescription drugs, and metabolic imbalances can all be mistaken for dementia.

- Alzheimer's disease is the cause of nearly 70% of all cases of true dementia. We don't know precisely what causes Alzheimer's disease, but decreased levels of acetylcholine seem to play a role.

- While Alzheimer's disease has no known cure, treatments are available that may temporarily reduce the symptoms or slow the process.

- Multi-infarct dementia, a series of small strokes in the brain that damage the parts associated with memory and other thought processes, is the second leading cause of dementia.

- Once your physician has ruled out conditions that would require more specific treatment, you might consider using ginkgo to alleviate symptoms of dementia.

Ginkgo and Memory

I n chapter 2, you read that all of us are prone to a worsening of memory as we get older. Although this age-associated memory impairment is normal, it certainly can be upsetting. The good news about normal age-associated memory loss is that not only is it very common, it also is quite possibly something that we can help. Some bad news, ironically, comes from these same features: because typical age-associated memory loss is a normal effect of aging and not a disease, it doesn't get much attention from medical researchers. Scientific studies on various treatments for memory loss almost always involve people with Alzheimer's disease or other severe forms of mental impairment.

As we'll see in this chapter, strong evidence shows that ginkgo can help protect memory and mental functioning in people with severe age-related mental decline. Later chapters will talk about other natural treatments as well as medications that have also been shown to be effective. But can these treatments help normal age-related memory loss?

The honest answer is that we don't know. The studies simply haven't been done.

Nonetheless, we have good reason to believe that ginkgo, phosphatidylserine, and other treatments for severe mental impairment may be useful for the merely annoying features of typical age-related memory loss. The thinking goes as follows: In the studies described below, ginkgo has proven helpful for improving mental function in both Alzheimer's disease and non-Alzheimer's forms of dementia. These diseases are very different in terms of what causes them and how they affect the brain. If ginkgo can have such a broad effect as this, then it makes sense that ginkgo might also be good for less serious kinds of memory impairment, such as ordinary age-associated memory loss.

Ginkgo is widely used in Germany as a medical treatment for ordinary age-related memory loss.

Such reasoning isn't proof, but it has been enough to convince many German physicians to prescribe ginkgo for normal age-related memory loss. It is widely used in North America by millions of people for the same purpose.

This chapter will describe what the research can tell us about ginkgo and severe memory impairment. Before we look at the research, though, we need to take a little detour and understand how researchers measure memory loss.

How Is Memory Measured?

How do you know when your memory is getting worse? Such changes are so gradual that often it is our loved ones who see the changes in our memory more clearly than we do ourselves. We all forget things from time to time—

phone numbers, the names of new acquaintances, or where we left our purse or wallet. Memory loss, however, means a subtle, slow *increase* in such everyday occurrences. How, then, can researchers measure something this hard to pin down? And how can doctors tell when a treatment for memory loss is working? This is not as difficult as it might sound.

In chapter 2, we discussed how different kinds of memories are actually stored in various areas of the brain. Our minds seem to process the memories of sights, sounds, and smells in different ways. To more effectively measure overall memory function, psychologists have developed a battery of tests for different types of memories.

One type of test measures *verbal* memory. A verbal test, for example, might feature a list of words that you are asked to read aloud. Then the list is put away, and you are asked to repeat all the words you can remember after this one reading.

As we mentioned in chapter 2, memory is strengthened by repetition. In a test such as this, the exercise would be repeated several times in a row to measure how your ability to remember the list improves.

The California Verbal Learning Test and the Rey Auditory Verbal Learning Test are two such tests for verbal memory. Other tests use computerized lists of names and grocery items to measure memory.[1] The Wechsler Memory Scale III uses stories and drawing tasks to measure both verbal and nonverbal memory. Other tests, such as the Alzheimer's Disease Assessment Scale (ADAS-Cog), are designed specifically to measure the severe memory impairment caused by a serious health condition.

Even with a variety of carefully designed tests, measuring relatively small or subtle changes in memory is not easy. From one day to the next, all of us experience small fluctuations in our memories, and for all kinds of reasons. Fatigue, stress, or illness, for instance, can make our

An Example of a Short-Term Memory Test

Read the following list aloud. Then put the list away, and see how many of the words you can correctly remember. Repeat this exercise a second and a third time, and see how many more words you can remember each time. This sample test is similar to verbal learning tests used by psychologists to measure memory.

apple	telephone
chair	spoon
bicycle	orange
refrigerator	light bulb
carpet	cheese
fan	cutting board
sofa	candle
teacup	

While this particular list has not been evaluated in studies, an informal survey revealed an average score of 4 the first time, 6 the next, and 9 items recalled after three readings.

memories suffer. However, severe memory impairment is easier to measure reliably than the gradual changes that accompany normal aging.

What Makes a Good Study?

Before we look at the ginkgo studies, I need to explain the basics of research in general. Once you understand this information, you'll be able to evaluate any medical research you read about in books or in the news, and you'll understand the rest of this chapter better.

What Is a Double-Blind Study?

Determining whether a treatment really works is not as easy as you might think. The biggest problem is the confusing influence of the power of suggestion. If I were to give you a sugar pill and tell you it would make you feel better, chances are good that you would feel better. This so-called placebo effect is surprisingly powerful. For some conditions, such as menopausal symptoms or prostate disease, placebo treatment can essentially make symptoms disappear in as many as 50% of people.[2]   While   nothing   is

The gradual changes in memory that come with age are difficult to measure reliably.

wrong with healing diseases with placebos (in fact, a lot is right with the method), this phenomenon makes it tricky to determine how well a treatment works in itself.

To get around this problem, researchers use the so-called *blinded placebo-controlled study.* Half the patients involved in the study are given real treatment (the treatment group), while the other half are given phony treatment (the placebo control group), and all patients are kept in the dark (they are "blind") about which group they are in. This technique factors out the power of suggestion. If the treatment group does better than the placebo control group, then researchers can conclude that the treatment really works.

It's also important to make sure that the doctor dispensing the pills doesn't know who is in which group. Doctors who are confident that they are giving a real treatment might unintentionally communicate this confidence to patients; this acts as the power of positive suggestion. They also tend to rate the results over-optimistically for the group they know is getting a medication. When both the doctor and the patient are in the dark, the experiment is considered a *double-blind* experiment. This way, the element of suggestion is eliminated. Generally speaking, we can trust only double-blind trials; we must consider the results of other types of studies contaminated by the mysterious power of the placebo effect.

Keeping the subjects "blind" is very important, but it can be tricky. For example, the smell and taste of a liquid preparation of some herbs is distinctive. Creating a substance that looks and tastes similar but has no active ingredients is difficult. This means that it's possible for those in the treatment group to know they are taking the real thing and for those in the control group to know they are taking a placebo. Similar problems occur in studies of conventional medications. If a treatment causes side effects, participants and physicians may be able to tell whether they are part of the treated group rather than the untreated (placebo) group. A reliable study will report on efforts to keep the subjects "blind."

Statistics Matter

We've said that only double-blind trials are reliable. However, there is one further requirement: *statistical significance.* This is a very important concept to understand when you read studies.

Sometimes you will read that people in the treatment group did better than those in the placebo group but that the results were not statistically significant. This means you cannot assume that the results proved the treatment was effective. Statistical significance is a mathematical technique used to ensure that the apparent improvement seen in the treated group represents a genuine difference, rather than just chance.

Consider the following analogy: Suppose you flip one coin 20 times and end up with 9 heads. Then, you flip a second coin 20 times and count 12 heads. Does this mean that the first coin is less likely to fall with the head side up than the second coin? Or was the difference just due to chance? A special mathematical technique can help answer this question. The bottom line is that when study results look good but aren't statistically significant, they can't be taken any more seriously than the apparent "bias" of the coin that happens to fall heads more often when you flip it a few times.

Studies on Ginkgo's Effectiveness

Now that you know what constitutes a good study, let's turn our attention to what the researchers have found regarding ginkgo's effects on our memories. Published reports from scientific research on this subject have been available since the mid-1980s. More than 40 scientific studies have evaluated ginkgo's effectiveness in treating memory loss and mental decline, nearly all of them focusing on relatively serious conditions such as Alzheimer's disease. The best of all these studies was published in 1997 in the *Journal of the American Medical Association (JAMA)*.

The Le Bars Study

This study, known as the Le Bars study after the principal author, makes a strong case that ginkgo extract can reduce symptoms of dementia caused by Alzheimer's disease or multi-infarct dementia. (As we saw in chapter 3, multi-infarct dementia is a dementia caused by a series of small strokes.) This influential double-blind placebo-controlled study obtained and analyzed data from more that 300 participants and followed over 200 of them for one full year.

Potential participants were accepted on the basis of examinations indicating that they had fairly severe mental impairment. Participants then received daily either 120 mg of a special ginkgo extract or an identical-looking placebo.

The ginkgo extract used in the Le Bars study was a semi-purified concentrate made from dried ginkgo leaves. Like most of the ginkgo products available on the market today, it was standardized to contain 24% flavonol glycosides and 6% terpenes. (See chapter 5 for more information on standardized ginkgo extracts.)

At 12, 26, and 52 weeks, the results of treatment were measured using three different tests. The first test, mentioned earlier in this chapter, evaluated memory and language skills. It is called the ADAS-Cog (short for *cognitive subscale* of the Alzheimer's Disease Assessment Scale). The second was an evaluation filled out by caregivers or family members. It is known as the GERRI scale (Geriatric Evaluation by Relative's Rating Instrument). The third test in the series reported the results of a structured interview conducted by a doctor and was designed to look at overall improvement. It is called the CGIC scale (Clinical Global Impression of Change).

Of the 309 participants of the Le Bars study, only 202 completed the year-long study. When such a significant number of people drop out of a study, statistical analysis is used to reduce any potential "bias" in the results. Such analysis was done for this study.

The memory and other mental tests in the ADAS-Cog revealed that, at the end of the study, 50% of the ginkgo group had improved compared to only 29% of the placebo group (see figure 4). The rest either remained the same or deteriorated further. Analysis of what caregivers noticed (the GERRI test) showed similar results: 37% of the patients taking ginkgo actually improved, while only 23% of the patients on the placebo improved (see figure 5). These differences were statistically significant.

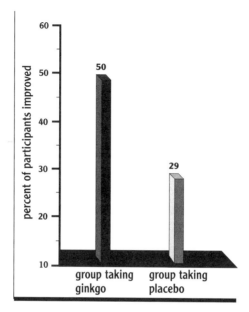

Figure 4. *Double-blind study (Le Bars, 1997) showed ginkgo improves memory and language skills (the ADAS-Cog test)*

The authors of the Le Bars study wondered whether these improvements were large enough to mean anything in "real life." To decide this, they looked at a large body of clinical knowledge about the ADAS-Cog test and concluded that a large improvement (4 points) on the ADAS-Cog "may be equivalent to a 6-month delay in the progression of the disease." It turned out that this level of improvement was found in 29% of the participants on ginkgo, compared to 13% on the placebo. The authors reported that this difference is about the same as that found in a high-dosage trial of tacrine, a medication prescribed for treatment of Alzheimer's (see chapter 10).

The CGIC (the structured interview conducted by doctors that measures overall improvement) didn't find

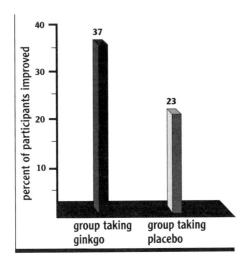

Figure 5. *The same study (Le Bars, 1997) showed caregivers notice more improvement in those given ginkgo than in those given placebo (the GERRI test)*

any difference. However, this wasn't a surprising result, as the CGIC scale only registers changes that are very large. In various studies, tacrine too has failed to influence CGIC scores while producing improvements on the ADAS-Cog. Neither ginkgo nor the approved drug tacrine appear to be powerful enough treatments to register on the CGIC scale.

So just what *does* the Le Bars study prove? It does *not* show that ginkgo is the magic potion to cure dementia. However, it did find that ginkgo can provide definite and meaningful benefits noticeable by caregivers and family members.

What the Le Bars study did *not* prove is also of some importance. Because this study used the same dose (120

A Major Study on Ginkgo's Effectiveness

A large and well-designed U.S. clinical trial on a special ginkgo extract was published by the prestigious *Journal of the American Medical Association* in 1997.[3] This study found that ginkgo stabilized, and in some cases improved, the mental and social functioning of patients with Alzheimer's disease as well as other forms of severe age-related mental decline. Changes were modest but large enough to be noticed by caregivers and family. The study's authors concluded that ginkgo extract "appears to stabilize and, in an additional 20% of cases (vs. placebo), improve the patient's functioning for periods of 6 months to 1 year."

Significantly, ginkgo did not appear to cause any side effects—at least no more than were found in the placebo group. Ginkgo extract is already widely used in Europe for treating age-related memory impairment. The publication of this study has helped accelerate the use of ginkgo extract here in North America.

mg a day) for all its participants, it tells us nothing about other doses. Would higher doses of ginkgo have helped more of the participants? Would higher doses have produced more improvement in any of the participants? Such questions await additional research.

Also, because it lasted only a year, the Le Bars study is also unable to address the issue of longer-term benefits. Finally, this study does not prove that ginkgo will help memory and mental function in people who are *not* suffering from dementia. But because Alzheimer's disease and multi infarct dementia have such different causes, and because ginkgo improved the mental functions of participants with *both* disorders, this study suggests that ginkgo might have an effect on many types of memory loss, including that caused by ordinary aging processes.

On a very positive note, participants who used ginkgo experienced almost no side effects. With the exception of some mild gastrointestinal upset, the adverse effects reported were the same for both the placebo and ginkgo groups.

The Kleijnen and Knipschild Review

As I mentioned earlier, the Le Bars study was not the only double-blind trial to look at the benefits of ginkgo in severe age-related mental decline. More than 40 clinical studies

In a major study, ginkgo appeared to stabilize and, in 20% of cases, to improve mental functioning in Alzheimer's patients.

have been performed in Europe. However, many of these were not as well designed as the Le Bars study. In 1992, Kleijnen and Knipschild critically reviewed all the double-blind ginkgo studies they could find that were performed up to that time.[4] They rated the quality of each study on a 100-point scale for seven different areas. The purpose was to determine which studies were performed well enough to be accepted as meaningful.

Trials receiving a total score of 65 or above were considered well performed. Only eight of the 40 studies reached this level. However, these eight studies involved a total of some 1,000 participants, a substantial number of people. For comparison purposes, the FDA might approve a typical prescription drug after studies involving a total of

1,000 to 2,000 persons showed that it was safe and effective. When you add in the Le Bars study and the two studies described below, a total of over 1,500 people have participated in properly designed studies of ginkgo for mental impairment. It is therefore fair to say that ginkgo as a treatment for Alzheimer's disease deserves to be taken seriously.

Most of the older studies described the enrolled participants using an outdated term: "cerebral insufficiency." This term dates back to the days when we thought mental decline was caused by marginally sufficient blood supply to the brain. Today, they would be categorized as suffering from Alzheimer's disease or non-Alzheimer's dementia.

A total of over 1,500 people have participated in properly designed studies of ginkgo for "cerebral insufficiency."

In the best of these studies, 99 patients were given either 150 mg per day of ginkgo extract or placebo. At the end of 12 weeks, 70% of the ginkgo group showed improvement, compared to 14% of the placebo group (see figure 6). Interestingly, these results are much more dramatic than what was seen in the Le Bars study. The reasons for this difference are unclear, but they may be due to the larger dose of ginkgo used.

The top eight clinical trials, their overall scores in the Kleijnen and Knipschild Review, the daily dose of ginkgo extract, the duration of each study, and the number of patients analyzed are presented in table 1. The ginkgo group fared better than the placebo group in each one of these studies.

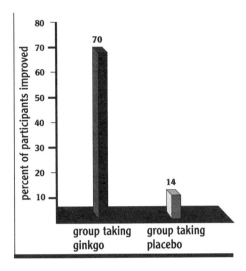

Figure 6. *Double-blind study shows participants taking ginkgo improved more than those given placebo* (Schmidt et al., 1991)

Since this 1992 review, two other well-designed double-blind studies performed in Europe have focused on the effectiveness of ginkgo. These involved a total of over 250 individuals with either Alzheimer's disease or multi-infarct dementia.[5,6] The largest of these enrolled 216 participants, and lasted for 6 months. Again, the results showed that ginkgo produced significant improvement in memory and mental function.

Putting all this research together, we can safely say that ginkgo improves memory, concentration, and alertness in individuals with Alzheimer's or non-Alzheimer's dementia.[7] Full effects appear to take at least 4 to 6 weeks to develop, and on average symptoms of poor mental performance are reduced about 25%.

Table 1. Clinical Trials Using Ginkgo for "Cerebral Insufficiency"

TRIAL	Ginkgo More Effective Than Placebo	Quality of study (0 - 100 scale)	Daily Dose	Duration of Treatment	No. Analyzed Ginkgo/Placebo
Schmidt et al. 1991[8]	Yes	90	150 mg	12 weeks	50/49
Brüchert et al. 1991[9]	Yes	80	150 mg	12 weeks	110/99
Meyer 1986[10]	Yes	80	4 mls (160 mg)	3 months	55/45
Taillandier et al. 1986[11]	Yes	80	160 mg	12 months	80/86
Haguenauer et al. 1986[12]	Yes	78	160 mg	3 months	34/33
Vorberg et al. 1989[13]	Yes	75	112 mg	12 weeks	49/47
Eckmann 1990[14]	Yes	67	160 mg	6 weeks	29/29
Wesnes et al. 1987[15]	Yes	67	120 mg	12 weeks	27/27

How Does Ginkgo Work?

Discovering *whether* a treatment works is often simpler than discovering *how* it works. We don't really know how most pharmaceutical treatments work. The same is true for ginkgo.

Ginkgo's full effects seem to take 4 to 6 weeks to develop.

We do know that ginkgo extract improves blood circulation[16] by thinning the blood and increasing the ability of red blood cells to fit through smaller spaces.[17] When blood cells are unable to fit into smaller spaces, this means they are less able to fit through the microscopic blood vessels known as capillaries. The capillaries bring blood and oxygen to the cells of our bodies. For many years, it was thought that mental functions declined because brain cells were getting less blood (and therefore, less food and oxygen). It was assumed that ginkgo improved mental function by increasing blood flow to the brain.

However, recent advances in science have challenged this understanding of mental impairment. Diminished blood flow is no longer considered the immediate cause of declining memory and mental function. A new generation of brain-scanning techniques have shown that there is *not* a direct connection between blood flow and thinking ability.

The primary problem in dementia appears to be cumulative damage to brain cells caused by a variety of influences. Increasing blood flow to the brain may help prevent *future* damage, thus slowing the progression of dementia. Researchers also point out that ginkgo may protect brain cells from damage through its *antioxidant* activity. Several studies, in fact, show that ginkgo is an effective antioxidant.[18–28]

However, there are many antioxidants. Ginkgo probably has a beneficial effect on dementia for *other* reasons besides its antioxidant properties. Ginkgo may stimulate nerve cells, or perhaps give them a chance to recover by protecting them from further injurious influences.[29] Considerable research is necessary before these questions can be answered with certainty.

Studies show that ginkgo is an effective antioxidant that can protect cells from damage.

There is one more question to answer with ginkgo: which of its constituents are responsible for the overall effects of the herb? Although we do not know the answer to this question, research has shown that the ginkgolide and flavonoid compounds in ginkgo have special properties, including the ability to inhibit blood platelet clumping. This action is thought to help protect against stroke damage as discussed in chapter 7.[30] However, assigning all of ginkgo's medicinal activity to the ginkgolides and the antioxidant flavonoids is quite possibly a mistake. Until we have further evidence, we can't assume that any of the components of ginkgo extracts are unimportant for the overall beneficial effects.

Ginkgo for Ordinary Age-Related Memory Loss

The above studies give us good reason to suspect that ginkgo may be helpful for ordinary age-related memory loss. As mentioned earlier, they suggest that ginkgo's effects on memory are general rather than specific. What I mean by this is that the effects aren't limited to people with Alzheimer's disease. Ginkgo appears to be effective in severe age-related memory loss and mental decline regard-less of the specific cause. For this reason, it seems logical to conclude that ginkgo has some type of general effect that might make it useful in a wide variety of circum-stances where memory or mental function are impaired.

Unfortunately, there has been very little research on ginkgo's effectiveness in people with ordinary memory loss. One small, double-blind placebo-controlled study ex-amined ginkgo's effects in eight healthy female volunteers, age 25 to 40, and found "very significant" improvements in short-term memory.[31,32] However, the number of par-ticipants in this study was far too small for it to be consid-ered reliable. Larger studies are needed before we can make any definite conclusions.

Despite the absence of hard evidence, health care practitioners are beginning to use ginkgo for ordinary age-related memory loss. For example, Richard Noble, M.D., of Portland, Oregon, regularly prescribes ginkgo for this condition. Gary, a patient in his mid-60s, was showing signs of significant loss of short-term memory. Dr. Noble placed him on ginkgo and then saw Gary and his wife for a follow-up exam several weeks later. While Gary didn't think he had improved much, his wife disagreed. She had noticed that Gary was definitely having an easier time finding such things as his glasses and his car keys.

Jill Stansbury, N.D., a naturopathic physician in Wash-ington, tells the story of an elderly woman patient in her 80s who complained of memory and balance problems. Dr. Stansbury prescribed standardized ginkgo extract tablets. "After taking the pills for 2 to 3 weeks, she got steadier on her feet and noticed improvements in her memory," Dr. Stansbury reported. "She kept this up for a few months and then quit. Six months later, her problems had returned." Treatment was once again resumed. "After 2 to 3 months of taking the pills the second time around, her problems cleared up again," explained Stansbury. But

Dr. Stansbury is quick to point out that ginkgo does not work for all her patients with dementia. Some who take it fail to benefit at all.

Michael Ancharski, N.D., of Tucson, Arizona, uses ginkgo for many of his patients over 60. One of them, a 70-year-old artist, had begun to forget important things. He would often go out in his car only to forget where he was going. He had even begun to leave paintings half-finished. After a few weeks of ginkgo, he appeared to be doing much better. His family reported that he no longer seemed so forgetful about his driving or his painting.

Andrew Rubman, N.D., tells of a 72-year-old retired university professor. This gentleman was concerned that he was losing the ability to quote entire paragraphs from his extensive library. This was something he had done in his classes for years, and he was very proud of this ability. The realization that his memory was slipping away caused him to feel depressed.

After taking ginkgo extract for less than 2 weeks, he seemed to be responding. Over time, the patient felt that he had regained 90% of his memory function and reported that his depression had returned to optimism.

Keep in mind that anecdotal reports such as these don't prove anything. We really need well-designed studies such as those described above. These reports do, however, help paint a picture of what kind of benefits you may be able to expect from ginkgo.

Ginkgo for Younger Adults

Thomas Kruzel, N.D., of Portland, Oregon reports that in his clinical experience ginkgo is even more helpful for younger adults than for older patients. Dr. Kruzel feels that he has gotten particularly good results working with school teachers. These patients are typically women in their 30s and 40s. They report that taking ginkgo helps them keep their mental processes together. They claim that ginkgo not only improves their memory but also their alertness, ability to think, and ability to deal with crises in the classroom. When taking ginkgo, these teachers reported that they were better able to meet the challenge presented by 25 demanding students, without experiencing what they called "brain fatigue" or burnout.

Such stories are intriguing, but again they are little more than testimonials. Without a control group and double-blind design, determining whether the apparent benefits reported by Dr. Kruzel are real or simply due to the power of suggestion is impossible.

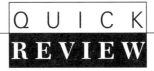

QUICK
REVIEW

- Strong evidence tells us that ginkgo can improve memory and mental function in people with dementia. A recent study of 300 people with Alzheimer's disease or non-Alzheimer's dementia reported in the *Journal of the American Medical Association* in 1997 found that ginkgo extract can slow the progression of Alzheimer's disease and non-Alzheimer's dementia and in some cases actually improve symptoms.

- Ten other well-designed studies, involving a total of over 1,200 participants, have also found that ginkgo can improve functioning in people suffering from memory impairment and related symptoms.

- It appears that ginkgo takes about 4 to 6 weeks to produce full benefits.

■ Virtually no research has been done on ginkgo's ability to help age-related memory loss in healthy people. However, it is logical to assume that ginkgo may have a general beneficial influence on memory, given that the herb works for such unrelated causes of dementia as Alzheimer's disease and multi-infarct dementia. Nonetheless, well-designed scientific studies are indispensable in the process of determining the effectiveness of a medication or herbal treatment.

How to Take Ginkgo

Now that you have read the evidence that ginkgo can improve memory and mental function, you may be interested in trying it yourself. Perhaps you have a loved one suffering from Alzheimer's disease or some other form of severe age-related memory loss, conditions for which there is strong evidence that ginkgo is effective. Or maybe you have ordinary age-related memory loss and want to try ginkgo to see whether it helps. In this chapter, you'll learn how much ginkgo to use, what kind to get, and how to take it. First, however, one caution: a medical evaluation is essential.

The Need for a Medical Evaluation

If you are thinking of suggesting ginkgo for a friend or relative with severe loss of mental function, or wish to use it yourself, please don't do so without first seeking medical advice. There may be a hidden medical illness causing the symptoms. If mental impairment were caused by side effects from prescription medications or a brain tumor, you certainly wouldn't want to just go ahead and recommend ginkgo. Obviously, the underlying condition needs to be treated!

If a physician does diagnose Alzheimer's disease or multi-infarct dementia, or ordinary age-related memory loss, then you may wish to consider ginkgo as a treatment. As we demonstrated in chapter 4, there is very good evidence that ginkgo can significantly improve memory and other aspects of mental function in people who have these diseases.

I would still recommend medical consultation before using ginkgo because there are certain standard medications that should not be combined with ginkgo. This issue is discussed further in chapter 6.

Dosage

The usual dose of ginkgo is 40 mg 3 times daily of a standardized extract, making a total of 120 mg a day. Higher doses—up to 240 mg a day—are sometimes recommended. We don't know, however, whether more is better, and higher doses may present greater risk of side effects.

In all the recent double-blind studies of ginkgo, the extract used was standardized to contain 24% flavonol glycosides and 6% terpene lactones.

Because the subject of herbal standardization is crucial and yet so little understood, I will take some time to explain it here.

Why Is a Standardized Extract Important?

When you purchase a drug, you know exactly what you are getting. Drugs are single chemicals that can be measured and quantified down to the molecular level. Thus a tablet of extra-strength Tylenol contains 500 mg of acetaminophen, no matter where or when you buy it. If generic Tylenol were found not to contain as much acetaminophen as was listed on the label, the manufacturer would be guilty of fraud. One bottle of acetaminophen should be just as good as any other. A simple chemical measurement can tell us this.

The usual dose of ginkgo is 40 mg 3 times daily of an extract standardized to 24% flavonol glycosides and 6% terpene lactones.

But the situation with herbs is much more complex. The main problem is that herbs don't contain just one chemical. Because they are living organisms, they produce hundreds or thousands of chemicals, in proportions that can vary from one plant to the next. Which ones should be listed on the label?

For ginkgo, as well as for many other herbs, we don't know for certain exactly which chemicals (and in what proportions) are responsible for all its helpful effects. We know that the flavonoids and terpenes are active ingredients, but further research is needed to completely understand their interactions and the contribution of all other constituents.

Because ginkgo's medicinal effect comes from a combination of many ingredients, and not from a single active ingredient, it actually makes sense to consider the total herbal product as the active material. Teasing apart the complete story of all the active ingredients and their interactions is simply not practical in the case of ginkgo and many other herbal products. As a result, we don't know which components matter most, and we have no easy way to compare the effectiveness of two ginkgo products.

Keep in mind that the exact components of an herb are influenced by such factors as the type of seed used,

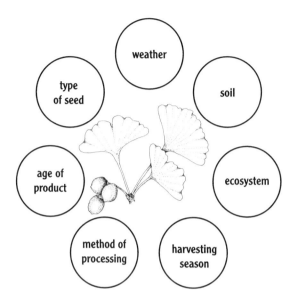

Figure 7. *The ginkgo you purchase is affected by many things*

the weather, the soil, the time of year the herb was harvested, where it was grown, the nature of nearby plants, the way the herb was processed, and how long the retail product sat on the shelf before purchase (see figure 7). The terpene concentration alone of dried ginkgo leaf material can vary by a factor of 40 between samples.[1] Simply put, when you purchase an herb, you face a lot of variables you don't have with drugs. This set of problems is a major reason why doctors are usually more comfortable prescribing drugs than herbs.

Modern European herbal companies have come up with a method that partially solves this problem. This process produces what is called a "standardized herbal extract." While it doesn't make herbs as interchangeable as batches of acctaminophen, it does go a long way toward making herbal products consistent. All the studies of ginkgo discussed in this book used standardized extracts, and it might be wise to choose a product of this type if you wish to try ginkgo.

A standardized extract is a concentrated herb preparation made by dissolving the herb in alcohol and water (or other solvents) and boiling it down until a certain fixed percentage of one or more key ingredients is reached. In some cases, including ginkgo, certain components are removed to more highly concentrate others.[2] The final product is said to be standardized to one or more chosen ingredients.

With ginkgo, extracts are standardized to their content of flavonol glycosides and terpene lactones. If the complete manufacturing process, from seed to shelf, includes all the controls necessary to guarantee a consistent final product, then we have good reason to believe that two batches of ginkgo prepared in this way are about equally effective.[3]

Most ginkgo products of this type are called 24/6 products, representing the 24% flavonol glycosides and 6% terpene lactones. The remaining 70% consists of other elements from ginkgo leaf (which may be very important).

Many 24/6 ginkgo products are available on the market today. They are either the actual European forms of ginkgo used in studies or products made in imitation of the European manufacturing methods. To make a pound of this type of ginkgo extract, you need about 50 pounds of ginkgo leaf. For this reason, such products also often say "50:1" on their labels.

Unfortunately, simply because a product is labeled 24/6 does not mean that it works the same as the ginkgo extracts found effective in double-blind studies. If two manufacturers use a different manufacturing process to produce ginkgo extract, their products may not be identical even if they both contain 24% flavonol glycosides and 6% terpenes. One problem is that there may be many other important ingredients in ginkgo that are not present in the same quantity in both products. Another possibility is that precisely which flavonol glycosides and terpenes are included could vary widely (there are many of them.)

Finally, be warned: Some manufacturers play a "numbers game" with ginkgo to try to sell their products. They list even higher percentages of flavonol glycosides and terpene lactones on the labels, hoping to give the impression that these products are thereby more powerful than other brands. This is simply marketing hype. Since we don't know all the active ingredients in ginkgo, we have no reason to believe that these higher-percentage products are more effective. In fact, they may even be less effective because the effort to increase the percentage of certain ingredients may reduce the presence of other unknown active ingredients. We should avoid falling into the trap of believing that higher numbers automatically mean a better product.

No clinical research data supports marketing suggestions that extracts standardized to a higher percentage than 24/6 make a better product.

It may be best to stick to products that have actually been subjected to clinical research. Your pharmacist or herbalist should be able to answer specific questions about the ginkgo product(s) they sell.

Other Forms of Ginkgo

Besides the usual 24/6 standardized extracts, a few other forms of ginkgo are also available. Keep in mind that "unstandardized" products may still work, even if they haven't been tested in clinical trials. Untested means *unproven*, which is different than *proven ineffective*. However, the only sure way to know that you are using a product that works is to choose one that has passed the test of well-designed clinical trials.

Some ginkgo products available on the market today are combined with soy phospholipids. The manufacturers state that this form is better absorbed than the usual standardized ginkgo. At present, however, we have no evidence that such products are better, or even that they work at all.

Another alternative to the usual standardized ginkgo extract is to try a simple alcohol tincture made from fresh or dry ginkgo leaves. Unlike a standardized extract, a tincture doesn't usually have a fixed percentage of flavonol glycosides and terpene lactones, and is not as concentrated.

Still other products contain only dried ginkgo leaves. Again, we have no idea whether they are effective. **Warning:** If you collect leaves from your neighborhood ginkgo tree in hopes of obtaining your own supply, make sure you do not use ginkgo seeds or fruit. These parts of the plant may present safety risks.

Finally, ginkgo products are often offered in combination. You can buy ginkgo with vitamins, ginkgo with other herbs, even ginkgo snack chips! Two herbs in particular—ginseng and gotu kola—are often featured in combination with ginkgo. Both of these herbs are sometimes said to improve mental functions, but there's little evidence for ginseng and essentially none at all for gotu kola. (See chapter 9 for information on ginseng.)

Overall, although I have myself used tincture of ginkgo, I recommend using standardized ginkgo extract. It is only that form of ginkgo for which we have scientific clinical evidence regarding effectiveness and safety.

Don't Give Up Too Soon

Remember that ginkgo is not fast acting. You may have to take ginkgo for several weeks before you experience any noticeable improvement in symptoms, and at least a couple of months for maximum effects. Improvements in memory, concentration, and thinking ability arise slowly and subtly—you don't wake up the next morning feeling like a genius. Sometimes you can only tell that ginkgo is working when you look back, or perhaps when your relatives or friends tell you that you have become less forgetful.

Apparently, ginkgo does not reverse the underlying cause of memory loss. It simply improves symptoms.

If you don't keep this in mind, you may quit too soon.

If a loved one is taking ginkgo for early dementia, you should notice some improvement in a month or two. Jennifer's uncle, for example, had reached the point where he could no longer remember what day it was. Every day he would ask someone. One day, after taking ginkgo for a couple of months, he said, "Today is Tuesday, isn't it?" and he was right.

Despite encouraging testimonials such as this one, don't expect miracles from ginkgo, or any other treatment for that matter. Ginkgo is useful but not magical. The research strongly suggests that ginkgo can slow the progress of Alzheimer's disease or multi-infarct dementia. It is logical to believe that it might also be helpful for normal age-related memory loss. But it's not realistic to look at ginkgo as a miracle cure. People who feel that ginkgo has helped them report some degree of improvement rather than a completely new brain!

Mary's Story

After Mary's 80-year-old grandmother was diagnosed with early Alzheimer's disease, Mary gave her some ginkgo. Alice tried it for one day and then declared, "It doesn't work." She refused to take it again.

Mary had done some reading and research about ginkgo and knew that you had to give it time. Alice was a strong-willed woman, though, and Mary knew she couldn't make her do anything she didn't want to do. After a couple of weeks Mary hit on a plan.

"Grandma," she said. "I really think you need to give that ginkgo a chance."

"Nope," she said. "I tried it and it didn't work."

"Grandma, do you remember when I was little and you were teaching me how to crochet?"

A big smile came over Alice's face. "You made a beautiful sweater. A red one."

Finally, keep in mind that ginkgo's effects fade when you stop taking it. Apparently, ginkgo does not reverse the underlying cause of memory loss. It simply improves symptoms.

When Not to Take Ginkgo

You should not take ginkgo for any memory loss or impairment of mental function that hasn't been evaluated first by a doctor. Memory loss can be a symptom of a serious health problem such as a chemical imbalance, a reaction to medication, or even a brain tumor or stroke. If you or a

"That's right," said Mary. "I kept it ever since." She pulled it out of a bag and handed it to the older woman.

Alice took it in her hands and turned it over.

"Grandma, do you remember what I did the first day we started crocheting together? How I got frustrated and tore it up?"

"Yes. You thought you should be able to make a sweater in five minutes," she said, half-lost in memory.

"Right. And do you remember what you told me?"

"Rome wasn't built in a day," they said, in unison.

"You kept telling me that the whole time I was growing up, Grandma. So now it's my turn. Please be a little more patient with the ginkgo."

Alice offered no more resistance. And ginkgo proved very helpful.

---

loved one seems to be showing signs of memory loss, see your doctor right away for an evaluation. Don't waste any time trying to treat yourself with ginkgo—you might have a treatable condition for which ginkgo would be useless.

As we'll see in chapter 6, ginkgo is generally safe. But if you are taking a blood-thinning medication, don't take ginkgo except under the supervision of your doctor. Ginkgo has a tendency to "thin" the blood and improve circulation. These sometimes beneficial properties may cause interactions with drugs such as warfarin (Coumadin), heparin, aspirin, pentoxifylline (Trental). Even natural products such as garlic, phosphatidylserine (PS), and high-dose vitamin E may conceivably cause problems, although none have been reported. See chapter 6 for more information on this important safety issue.

Don't Forget to Treat the Whole Person

In our pill-happy society, we often look for quick fixes to complicated problems. This is understandable—who wouldn't rather get rid of a problem as quickly as possible? But the quick-fix method is not as successful in the long term as is a holistic approach—that is, one that treats the whole person.

Memory loss may have many causes. It seems likely that numerous factors affect memory, including diet, stress, personal habits, and other lifestyle issues. It's important, therefore, to take all these factors into account and not just focus on ginkgo. Later chapters in this book will discuss exercises that can help to sharpen your memory, as well as other natural treatments you can try. Also, you should think about your health in general. By eating well, getting moderate exercise, and reducing stress in your life, you'll be giving any treatment you try the best possible chance to help you.

Combining ginkgo with blood-thinning medications can be dangerous.

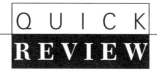

- If you want to use ginkgo to treat memory loss, you should first get a medical diagnosis to rule out a treatable underlying problem.

- The typical dosage of ginkgo is 120 mg per day of an extract standardized to contain 24% flavonol glycosides and 6% terpene lactones.

- Ginkgo typically takes weeks to produce results and a couple of months or more to reach its full effect.

- Because of ginkgo's blood-thinning properties, combining it with blood-thinning medications could be dangerous. See chapter 6 for a detailed discussion of safety issues regarding ginkgo.

- Ginkgo should be used as part of a holistic treatment plan that addresses diet, lifestyle, and other factors in a person's life.

Safety Issues

When it comes to treatment, safety is as important as effectiveness. Whether you are using an herbal product or an over-the-counter medication, finding something that actually *works* is important, but it is also vital that the treatment be safe. Most medications have side effects, some of which can be serious. Natural products are no exception. Before you take any medication, you should evaluate the benefits against the possible risks. Side effects, toxicity, drug interactions, and long-term safety are all aspects of safety that must be considered.

While drugs must undergo extensive formal study for their safety and effectiveness, herbs do not undergo the same type of scrutiny in the United States. From a legal point of view, they are simply regarded as a special category of food. Not only are they exempt from safety testing prior to marketing, but herbal medicine manufacturers, unlike prescription drug manufacturers, are not required to track and report adverse side effects that occur after the product is available. For this reason, we do not know as much as we would like about how well herbs work and any risks they may present.

However, the form of ginkgo used today first became available in Germany, where herbs do receive considerable scrutiny. Furthermore, thousands of people have been given ginkgo in formal clinical trials where safety issues were carefully considered. For this reason, we have more information regarding its safety than we do for most other herbs. The cumulative evidence suggests that ginkgo causes few side effects at normal doses and is not very toxic even when taken in excessive doses (at least in animals). However, there are few safety precautions that may be advisable when you use ginkgo. This chapter will tell you what we know and don't know about ginkgo's safety.

The Difference Between Side Effects and Toxicity

Most people have suffered side effects—unpleasant, unintended consequences—when using a medication. Some occur only rarely; others regularly accompany the use of certain products. Many over-the-counter antihistamines frequently cause fatigue and mental cloudiness, and decongestants commonly cause insomnia. Certain antibiotics lead to yeast infections so reliably that doctors often prescribe anti-yeast treatment right from the start.

Side effects can occur with almost any substance, even foods. Dairy products may produce mucous congestion, and beans and legumes can cause bloating and gas. It is no surprise, therefore, that herbs can cause side effects too.

Annoying side effects may occur at normal or even low doses of a treatment, but they generally go away when you stop using whatever caused them. We usually use a different word—*toxicity*—to refer to more serious adverse effects including permanent injury to the body. Most

Balancing Benefit Against Risk

Balancing the side effects of a treatment against the threat of an illness is important. With a life-threatening condition, physicians are more willing to accept a higher level of risk in the treatment.

We can see this process at work with cancer chemotherapy. Such treatments are highly toxic. However, when you're combating a life-threatening illness such as cancer, such measures make sense. Using a harsh treatment may well be worth the risk if the other choice is imminent death.

On the other hand, treating a common cold with a drug that could cause serious harm wouldn't make much sense. The cure might be worse than the illness.

commonly, toxic reactions occur when a substance is taken in excessive doses.

To understand the difference, compare the drugs Prozac and acetaminophen. At normal dosages, Prozac can cause insomnia, headache, nausea, sexual problems, and other unpleasant side effects. If you were to take 20 Prozac pills, however, it is likely that nothing serious would happen to you. In other words, Prozac causes numerous side effects but is not very toxic.

Acetaminophen, on the other hand, seldom causes any side effects when taken at the proper dosage. If you take too much acetaminophen, though, you are likely to suffer severe or even fatal liver damage. Thus acetaminophen causes few side effects but is potentially toxic.

The good news about ginkgo is that it appears to be quite safe from both these perspectives.

Whenever you are deciding whether to use a treatment, you have to balance the risk and the benefit. This issue comes up with ginkgo as well. Alzheimer's disease is so devastating that even a risky treatment might be worth trying. However, if you wish to use ginkgo for ordinary age-related memory loss, you need to make very sure that you are not potentially incurring more harm than benefit.

Fortunately, ginkgo seems to be safe enough that the decision isn't that difficult. There doesn't appear to be much of a down side when ginkgo is used appropriately. (See chapter for specific situations in which you should avoid taking ginkgo.)

Ginkgo's Excellent Side-Effect Profile

Extensive evidence suggests that ginkgo causes very few side effects. In the review of 40 studies discussed earlier, side effects occurred no more often in the groups that took ginkgo than in those that took the placebo.[1] (Yes, even people given placebo complain of a certain percentage of side effects! The power of suggestion works both ways.) When a treatment produces no more side effects than a placebo, it seems reasonable to say that it is side-effect free. And there were no *serious* side effects at all. Another review of nearly 10,000 participants taking ginkgo extracts in clinical trials showed that less than 1% experienced any side effects, and those that did occur were minor, such as mild digestive distress, headaches, and dizziness.[2]

Ginkgo certainly appears to cause fewer side effects than standard medications used for Alzheimer's disease. A German review of over 12,000 patients taking either ginkgo or standard medications found that patients taking medications reported about three times as many side effects as did those taking the herb.[3] However, such a comparison is rather informal. Only studies in which participants take either one treatment or another can give us a truly trustworthy side-effects comparison.

When a treatment produces no more side effects than a placebo, it seems reasonable to say that it is side-effect free.

Keep in mind that all these studies involved standardized ginkgo leaf extract, as described in chapter 5. We don't know much about the safety of fresh or dried ginkgo leaf, and we do know that ginkgo fruit and seeds can cause various problems.

Toxicity

While a given drug may have few side effects at a normal dose, it can be toxic if taken in excess. Because it would be unethical to overdose human subjects to determine toxic effects, scientists usually evaluate the toxicity of potential treatments by testing them in mice, rats, and other laboratory animals. The results of these studies are reported as the LD_{50}, the dose that it takes to kill half of the test animals (lethal dose 50%). If a substance passes animal testing with a high LD_{50}, then it is considered likely to be relatively safe in humans.

Toxicity is an important factor to consider when weighing treatment options. Many commonly used medications, such as the heart medication digitalis, can cause toxic (sometimes lethal) effects at doses not far above their usual therapeutic doses. If you accidentally double your dose of digitalis, you should probably call 911.

The good news about ginkgo is that animal studies have shown it to be quite non-toxic. Researchers could not find a toxic dose for ginkgo extract in rats, while the amount of extract lethal to half the test mice was found to be 7.73 mg for each *gram* of weight of the mouse.[4] Scaled up to our size, this toxic dose of ginkgo would mean more than *one pound* of extract for a 150-pound person, a staggering 8,780 capsules, 60 mg each, of ginkgo extract!

The toxic dose of ginkgo in mice, scaled up to our size, would equate to a 150-pound person ingesting 8,780 capsules, 60 mg each, of ginkgo extract.

While it's always possible that a particular individual will show an unusual reaction to ginkgo, overall the safety studies with ginkgo extract indicate that it is a very safe treatment.

However, one possible risk needs to be addressed: bleeding.

Ginkgo and Bleeding

Ginkgo makes the blood less likely to form clots. This effect is often informally described as "thinning" the blood and makes ginkgo a potentially useful treatment for several conditions, such as heart disease. Aspirin is believed to prevent heart attacks by reducing the chance of a clot forming in the arteries of the heart. However, blood-thinning treatments can cause problems too. Aspirin, for example, can be dangerous for people with a tendency toward internal bleeding. According to a few case reports, ginkgo may present similar risks.

One reported case involved a 33-year-old woman who had been taking ginkgo extract for 2 years.[5] She developed bleeding in the skull. Following successful treatment, it was experimentally determined that her blood was taking longer to clot while she was on ginkgo than after she stopped. Another case also involved bleeding in the skull.[6] This time the patient was a 72-year-old woman who had been taking ginkgo extract.

While we can't tell for sure whether ginkgo was the cause of the problem in these two cases,[7] they are certainly somewhat worrisome. Nonetheless, keep in mind that internal bleeding occurs sometimes by itself. Furthermore, internal bleeding was not observed among the thousands of people who took ginkgo in clinical trials. Most likely, if ginkgo causes bleeding at all, it does so rarely (when used by itself—see the next section for possible problems when treatments are combined). However, people with a known tendency to bleed more easily should not use ginkgo except under medical supervision. Furthermore, ginkgo should not be used before or immediately after surgery or during labor and delivery, because those are two situations in which you don't want to bleed any more than you have to.

Drug Interactions

Even if ginkgo by itself seldom (if ever) causes bleeding, there is one situation in which the risk may be higher: when ginkgo is combined with drugs or other substances that themselves thin the blood. Even the mild blood-thinning effects of ginkgo could be enough to raise the tendency to bleed too far when it is taken in such combinations.

There is one case report of bleeding in the iris of the eye in a 70-year-old man who was taking both ginkgo and aspirin.[8] The possibility of an interaction between aspirin and ginkgo makes sense because aspirin is known to thin the blood.

You might ask this question: If ginkgo can cause problems when combined with aspirin, why didn't any bleeding problems develop in all the thousands of people who participated in ginkgo studies in Germany? Surely some of them took aspirin! However, in most of those studies, participants were required not to take any blood-thinning medication, so the absence of bleeding seen in those studies tells us nothing about possible drug interactions.

Ginkgo's blood-thinning effect is a significant concern, as many people in the same age group that might use ginkgo also take blood-thinning drugs. The bottom line is this: *If you are taking any medication that affects the ability of the blood to clot, you should not take ginkgo except on the advice of your physician.* Such drugs include warfarin (Coumadin), heparin, pentoxifylline (Trental), and aspirin. It is also conceivable that natural substances with slight blood-thinning effects could cause problems when combined with ginkgo, such as garlic, phosphatidylserine (PS), and high dose vitamin E, although no such cases have been reported.

If you take a blood-thinning drug such as warfarin (Coumadin), pentoxifylline (Trental), heparin, or aspirin, consult your physician before taking ginkgo.

Long-Term Safety

It's always much more difficult to discover long-term dangers of treatments than immediate problems. Considering how many millions of people have taken ginkgo, any problems

Ginger's Story

Ginger was a 72-year-old woman who definitely didn't have Alzheimer's disease. She was the leader of a book club, a member of an amateur theatrical company, and a frequent contributor to the local newspaper. However, she was troubled by gaps in her memory. "I have to write everything down or it flies right out of my brain," she said. "Well, not *everything.* I can remember books I like just fine, and I can keep track of my lines, but if I go to the store without making a list, I'll forget half the things I planned to get."

She came to me wondering whether she should try ginkgo. I planned to explain to her that ginkgo had not been proven effective for people with mild memory loss, but might in fact be helpful anyway. However, before I could get to this she pulled out a bottle of pills and showed them to me. "These are my medications," she said.

One struck my eye immediately. It was labeled "warfarin sodium," the generic name for Coumadin.

that develop rapidly would probably have been noticed by now. Long-term risks, however, can be very difficult to identify. The hormone estrogen is a good example. Many millions of women take it and feel fine. But there is good evidence that it may cause an increased risk of breast cancer when taken for a long time. Individuals using a treatment such as estrogen cannot observe this type of long-term harm. You need formal studies involving thousands of participants that last for many years. Unfortunately, this has not been done for ginkgo (nor for many standard pharmaceuticals).

"Why are you taking this one?" I asked. It turned out that she suffered from atrial fibrillation, a form of heart arrhythmia that can create blood clots. Her cardiologist felt that she needed to take Coumadin to avoid the risk of stroke.

I shook my head and said, "I wouldn't take ginkgo right now if I were you. Whenever you take Coumadin, you are running the risk of internal bleeding. With careful attention, the drug can be used safely, but ginkgo might tip the balance. Consider it this way," I said. "You are doing fine now. Your memory problems are no more than an annoyance. Why risk catastrophe?" She agreed after I explained the reasons.

But that wasn't the end of the story. Two years later she came back to tell me that she was seeing a new cardiologist who had taken her off Coumadin. At this point I felt it was safe for her to try ginkgo.

—Steven Bratman, M.D.

While ginkgo has been widely used in Europe for nearly 2 decades and no harmful effects have been reported, this doesn't rule out the possibility that there are hidden, subtle, or occasional side effects that simply haven't been noticed. Therefore, in the absence of long-term studies, it is impossible to say with certainty that ginkgo is safe over the long term.

Some people feel that because ginkgo is a natural herb, it's likely to be safer in the long run than a drug. This, however, is an emotional rather than a rational statement. A few herbs have been shown to have long-term, or chronic, toxic potential, such as comfrey root. In other words, there is no guarantee that ginkgo is safe just because it's natural.

In fact, the same lack of knowledge prevails for many of today's most prescribed medications. The only absolutely foolproof way to determine whether or not long-term harm exists would be to take two identical populations, give one half the drug and the other half the placebo, and keep the experiment going for decades. If after 50 years or so no problems appeared in the treated group and their offspring, you could then conclude that a treatment was absolutely safe in the long run. Obviously, such a study has never been done, whether for drugs, herbs, vaccinations, food preservatives, or foods.

There is, however, one way to gather meaningful information about the long-term safety of a treatment. If you give an herb or drug to a rat for 6 months' duration, that equates roughly to giving it to a person for 20 years or more. Such research has been performed for ginkgo. According to studies involving rats, dogs, and rabbits, long-term use of ginkgo does not cause any detectable harm.[9] In particular, no adverse effects were seen in either reproductive function or in the health of offspring. While this is not an absolute guarantee of long-term safety in humans, it is definitely reassuring.

Is Ginkgo Safe During Pregnancy and While Nursing?

There have been no tests or studies conducted on the use of *Ginkgo biloba* by pregnant or nursing mothers. Considering this conspicuous lack of evidence, those who are pregnant, trying to get pregnant, or are currently nursing would do best to avoid it.

Is Ginkgo Safe for Children?

Perhaps this question should really be "why would children be taking ginkgo?" The answer, as you might guess, is that they don't really need to. All the well-documented uses of ginkgo are for conditions that only develop with age. Children, especially very young children, can be much more sensitive than adults; they can develop problems with treatments that cause no trouble at all for adults.

However, according to Steven Bratman, M.D., many parents have tried ginkgo as a substitute for Ritalin (a medication for treating attention deficit disorder). He specifically recalls one set of parents who gave their child ginkgo so she would remember to do her chores!

It probably isn't a good idea to give ginkgo to children. Its safety has not been established, and furthermore, it is not at all likely to get the chores done!

Is Ginkgo Safe for Those with Liver or Kidney Disease?

Virtually all substances we take in are "processed" by the liver and the kidneys. People with diseases of these organs almost always have to exercise particular caution using drugs of any kind. Herbal products are no exception. If you or your loved one has a disease or disorder of the kidneys or liver, consulting with your family physician before using ginkgo is important.

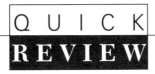

- Extensive evidence indicates that ginkgo is a safe treatment when used correctly.

- Ginkgo does not appear to produce any more side effects than placebo. Occasionally, people report some minor problems such as mild nausea, headaches, upset stomach, diarrhea, and dizziness.

- In animal studies, even large overdoses of ginkgo caused no detectable harm.

- The only real safety concerns regarding ginkgo relate to possible bleeding problems. Because ginkgo "thins" the blood, it should not be used by people with a tendency toward bleeding, except on a physician's advice. Ginkgo should also not be used before or immediately after surgery, or during labor and delivery. Finally, there may be problems when ginkgo is combined with blood-thinning medications such as warfarin (Coumadin), heparin, pentoxifylline (Trental), or aspirin. It is also conceivable that ginkgo might cause problems if combined with natural products that slightly thin the blood, such as garlic, phosphatidylserine (PS), and high dose vitamin E.

- The safety of using ginkgo over the long term has not been proved, although animal studies suggest that it is safe.

- Ginkgo's safety has not been proven for young children, women who are pregnant or nursing, or for those with severe kidney or liver disease.

Other Uses of Ginkgo

lmost all the scientific evidence for the use of
ginkgo relates to its effects on memory and mental
function. However, both doctors and researchers
have recommended ginkgo as a treatment for other conditions as well. This chapter briefly looks at some of these
additional uses of ginkgo. Many are based on ginkgo's ability to increase blood circulation, as discussed in previous
chapters.

Please keep in mind that some of the conditions you'll
read about in this chapter can be quite serious themselves, or may be caused by a serious underlying problem.
Do not attempt to use ginkgo as substitute for comprehensive medical care.

Intermittent Claudication

Intermittent claudication is a cramp-like pain and weak-
ness in the legs caused by an insufficient supply of oxygen.
It occurs after mild exercise and limits the ability to walk

distances. In severe cases, it becomes impossible to walk a full city block. The underlying cause of intermittent claudication is atherosclerosis (hardening of the arteries). In severe atherosclerosis, plaque blockades major arteries going to the leg muscles and prevents enough oxygen from reaching them.

The bottom line is this: Ginkgo extract appears to reduce the symptoms of intermittent claudication, producing measurable if not dramatic improvements in the ability to walk distances.

Obviously, the best approach to this condition is prevention. Stopping smoking, reducing blood pressure, controlling cholesterol levels, and making other healthful lifestyle changes are the most important steps you can take. For more information on what you can do to prevent atherosclerosis and all the diseases that it causes, see *The Natural Pharmacist Guide to Heart Disease Prevention.*

Intermittent claudication is difficult to treat. The most common treatment for severe blockage is surgery. The procedure transplants healthy blood vessels to form a "bypass" around the blockages in the legs. This approach is a long-term solution only when the underlying causes are eliminated as well. Without lifestyle changes, the transplanted vessels will eventually become blocked all over again.

Sometimes physicians will try using the medication Trental (pentoxifylline) to alleviate symptoms and postpone surgery. It makes blood flow more easily and may reduce symptoms to some extent. Doctors and patients have tried ginkgo as well, based on its known effects on blood circulation. A recent double-blind placebo-controlled study evaluated the benefits of ginkgo in 111 individuals with intermittent claudication.[1] Subjects were measured for pain while walking up a 12° slope on a treadmill. At the beginning of treatment, both the placebo and ginkgo group were able to walk only about 350 feet without pain. At the end of the trial, both groups had improved significantly (again, the power of placebo is amazing!). However, the ginkgo group had improved more: They were able to walk an average of 500 feet without pain, compared to 415 feet for the control group. This improvement was not miraculous, but it was still significant.

Positive results were seen as well in another recent double-blind placebo-controlled study.[2] At least 15 studies published through 1991 also found ginkgo helpful, although only two were of acceptable scientific quality.[3]

The bottom line is this: Ginkgo extract appears to reduce the symptoms of intermittent claudication, producing measurable if not dramatic improvements in the ability to walk distances. For other natural treatments that may help intermittent claudication, see *The Natural Pharmacist: Your Complete Guide to Illnesses and Their Natural Remedies.*

PMS Symptoms

During the week or so prior to their menstrual periods, many women develop uncomfortable bloating, swelling, and other signs of fluid retention, often in association with other PMS symptoms. In 1993, two French researchers published the results of a double-blind study that found ginkgo effective for the treatment of these so-called congestive symptoms.[4] They also examined gingko's effects on other PMS symptoms that they felt might be related to fluid buildup, such as headache and irritability.

The study evaluated 143 women, 18 to 45 years of age, and followed them for two menstrual cycles. All women admitted to the study had experienced PMS-related congestive symptoms for at least three consecutive cycles.

Jeanette's Story

Jeanette, a 67-year-old-woman, had been physically fit most of her life, though she was a heavy smoker.

Because she enjoyed walking, Jeanette did most of her errands on foot or by bus. After two years of easily walking to and from stores and the bus stop, she began to experience pain in her legs. The pain progressed to the point that she found it difficult to go two blocks to a supermarket. At her best friend's urging, she made an appointment with her longtime doctor (her son drove her to the office) and explained the problem. It didn't take him long to diagnose intermittent claudication.

When the study began, each woman received either the ginkgo extract or a placebo on day 16 of the first cycle. Treatment was continued until the fifth day of the next cycle, and resumed again on day 16 of that cycle.

The results were impressive. As compared to placebo, ginkgo significantly relieved major symptoms of fluid accumulation, particularly breast pain.

Although this was only one study, it was reasonably large, and the results deserve to be taken seriously. If additional research confirms these results, ginkgo may soon become widely accepted as a treatment for PMS.

For other natural treatments that may help PMS, see *The Natural Pharmacist Guide to PMS.*

Macular Degeneration

Impaired blood circulation to the sensitive eye tissue called the macula is thought to be a contributing factor to the condition known as macular degeneration. Since

"This is only the first shot over the bow," he said. "If the arteries in your legs are this clogged, your heart can't be in good shape either. You have to stop smoking." Jeanette decided to finally take his advice about smoking. It was quite difficult to quit, but his other suggestion was easy: take ginkgo.

After a few months, she found she was able to walk to the store and bus stop. A small victory for Jeanette, but an important one in restoring her sense of independence.

ginkgo can promote blood flow, it has been proposed as a possible treatment for this serious condition.

The macula is the part of the retina that produces the clearest vision, and degeneration of the macular tissue is a major cause of blindness in the elderly. Macular degeneration actually comes in two forms. One form, known as wet or *neovascular* macular degeneration, can be treated surgically with excellent results. The more common type, dry or *atrophic* macular degeneration, does not respond well to any form of standard medical treatment.

Ginkgo may offer some benefit for this second type of macular degeneration, although the evidence is weak. The only

Ginkgo may offer some benefit for the more common atrophic macular degeneration, but the direct evidence is weak.

direct evidence we have is one small double-blind study in which ginkgo extract appeared to improve long distance vision in people with macular degeneration.[5]

Warning: Do not try to use ginkgo for the first type of macular degeneration in lieu of surgery. You may needlessly lose your sight.

Other Vision Problems

Ginkgo has been proposed as a treatment for various vision problems associated with diabetes, such as cataracts and retinopathy. For these conditions, researchers have focused more on its antioxidant effects than on its blood-thinning abilities. However, the only direct evidence that ginkgo might be helpful comes from animal studies.[6,7] Research needs to be done in people before ginkgo can be considered a proven treatment for diabetic vision problems.

Ringing in the Ears (Tinnitus)

Ringing in the ears can be an extremely annoying problem, and in the majority of the cases, no treatable cause can be found. Since impaired blood flow may be a cause in some cases of tinnitus, ginkgo has been suggested as a possible treatment. However, there has not been much research to establish that it works.

One study suggests that ginkgo may relieve the symptoms of tinnitus,[8] while others have found it to be ineffective.[9,10] One of the negative studies used too low a dose of ginkgo and for too short a time to possibly work. The other enrolled only people with severe, long-standing tinnitus, while the positive study involved people who had just started to develop ringing in the ear. It is probably most accurate to say that we don't yet know whether ginkgo is effective for certain forms of tinnitus, but that it certainly deserves more study.

Impotence

Impaired circulation can cause symptoms of impotence. For this reason, ginkgo has been tried as a treatment. The results, however, are not yet conclusive. In one study, 50 men under the age of 70 suffering from impotence were treated with ginkgo extract for 6 months. The men who were able to achieve an erection from drug injection (this was before Viagra was available) regained spontaneous erections after treatment with ginkgo extract as well. Of the 30 men who did not previously respond to drug injections, 19 were helped and 11 remained impotent.[11]

Although these results are encouraging, I am not about to begin touting ginkgo as an effective alternative to Viagra. Because this study had no placebo group, it's not possible to tell how much of the benefit seen was due to the power of suggestion. Numerous studies have found that the placebo effect is enormously powerful in impotence. As always, properly designed double-blind studies are necessary.

An interesting new potential use of ginkgo has just come to the fore at press time: using ginkgo to treat the sexual side effects caused by antidepressant medications. One of the big problems with medications such as Prozac is that they can cause impotence in men and inability to achieve orgasm in women. The possibility that ginkgo may be able to help first came to light accidentally when an older patient on antidepressant medication tried ginkgo for memory enhancement, and reported improved erections.

In an open study that followed, 33 women and 30 men suffering from antidepressant-induced sexual dysfunction were given about 240 mg of extract a day. (Again, there was no placebo group.) An impressive 91% of the women and 76% of the men reported positive results.[12] While these results are quite promising, properly designed double-blind studies are necessary to establish whether ginkgo is really an effective treatment for this condition.

Depression

Depression is the number one mental health problem affecting the elderly. It is also a common feature of certain kinds of dementia. Researchers have noted that elderly people treated with ginkgo extract for dementia often be-

Ginkgo may be effective in treating depression, but well-designed tests are necessary to prove this benefit.

came less depressed. This observation has given rise to the idea that ginkgo may be effective in treating depression per se.

One placebo-controlled study directly evaluated whether ginkgo alleviated symptoms of depression.[13] The study consisted of 40 individuals over the age of 50 who had all failed to respond well to standard antidepressants. Half were given 80 mg of ginkgo extract 3 times a day *along with their regular antidepressant med-*

ications. The other half were given a placebo. The results showed that ginkgo was significantly helpful at improving symptoms of depression.

Taken along with the results seen in people with dementia, this study has led to the idea that ginkgo might be a useful general antidepressant for people over 50. However, this was only a preliminary study, and in any case it does not tell us whether ginkgo produces antidepressant effects when taken alone (rather than combined with standard treatments). Further study is necessary.

For more information on natural treatments for depression, see *The Natural Pharmacist Guide to St. John's Wort and Depression.*

Strokes and Heart Attacks

Ginkgo's ability to increase blood flow may make it useful in preventing and treating strokes and heart attacks. As we mentioned in chapter 3, strokes occur when arteries in the brain become blocked. The cells "downstream" of the blockage are left without a supply of blood. The result is that they are either severely damaged or die. This lack of oxygen causes what is known as "ischemic damage," and it can cause serious injury to entire areas of the brain. Heart attacks are quite similar.

It has been suggested that ginkgo may help prevent this damage by improving blood flow. While this has not yet been proven, there is some evidence that ginkgo can prevent another kind of damage that occurs later following a stroke or heart attack. What happens is this: After the immediate blockage and death of downstream tissues, the blockage soon decreases to some extent, and blood flow returns to the previously oxygen-starved areas. Like heavy rain after a drought, the return of the blood can cause its own form of injury, known as oxidative damage. The effects can be as bad as those of the original injury caused by the lack of oxygen.

In animal studies, ginkgo has been shown to reduce this type of injury.[14] For this reason, as well as its known influence on blood flow, medical practitioners have suggested that ginkgo extract may be helpful in preventing multi-infarct dementia, strokes, and the subsequent damage caused by these events. However, this has not been proven.

Preliminary evidence suggests that ginkgo may be helpful in related conditions, such as spinal cord injury[15] and heart attacks.[16,17] It is not clear which chemical compounds in ginkgo account for these actions. Various studies have pointed to ginkgolides,[18] flavonoids,[19] or yet another compound in ginkgo.[20]

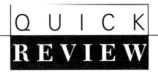

- Ginkgo is used for other purposes in addition to treating age-related decline of memory and mental function. Please note that some of the conditions discussed in this chapter can be quite serious themselves, or may be caused by a serious underlying problem. Do not attempt to use ginkgo as a substitute for comprehensive medical care.

- Probably the best studied of ginkgo's other uses is for the painful condition known as intermittent claudication. A few properly performed clinical trials have found that ginkgo extract can increase pain-free walking distance.

- One double-blind study suggests that ginkgo can reduce symptoms of PMS related to fluid congestion, particularly breast tenderness.

- Much weaker evidence suggests that ginkgo may be helpful for impotence, sexual side effects of antidepressant medications (inability to achieve orgasm in women, impotence in men), tinnitus, depression, "dry" macular degeneration and other vision problems. It may also be helpful for preventing and treating strokes and heart attacks, but much more research needs to be done.

Phosphatidylserine for Memory

P hosphatidylserine, or PS, has been hailed as "the brain nutrient." One best-selling book even claims that it "rejuvenates" brain cells and "charges up cell membranes." If you've heard the buzz about PS, you're probably wondering how much is fact and how much is fiction. While some of the claims for PS are exaggerated, don't let that discredit this useful supplement. Evidence from good clinical trials supports the use of PS in severe memory loss and mental impairment.

PS has been widely used in Italy and other parts of Europe since at least the mid-1980s. Lately, interest in the supplement has been growing on this side of the Atlantic too. Just as with ginkgo, nearly all the scientific evidence for PS relates to conditions of severe mental impairment, such as Alzheimer's dementia. However, it is logical to surmise that PS may be beneficial for ordinary age-related memory loss as well.

What Is PS and Where Does It Come From?

Phosphatidylserine (fos-fah-TIDE-ul-ser-een) is a member of a class of chemical compounds known as *phospholipids.* Part fatty acid and part phosphate, this substance is a component of the natural makeup of our bodies. Our diets do not provide much PS. It is synthesized from scratch in the body.

If you've heard the buzz about PS, you may be wondering how much of it is fact and how much is fiction.

PS is an essential component in all our cells; specifically, it is a major component of the cell membrane. The cell membrane is a kind of "skin" that surrounds living cells. Besides keeping cells intact, this membrane performs vital functions such as moving nutrients into cells and pumping waste products out of them. PS plays a vital role in many of these functions.

There are particularly high concentrations of PS in brain cells. In chapter 2, we described how our nervous system is composed of *neurons* interconnected to form a vast network of electrochemical communication. In the brain, our thoughts and memories are transmitted along these circuits as electrical messages. These signals travel along the network of neurons, hopping from one to the next.

Neurons are long cells. When information enters one end of a neuron, it has to travel some distance to get to the other end. The cell membrane of the neurons plays a major role in this signal transmission. Because PS is one of the major components of nerve cell membranes, it at least indirectly plays an important role in transmitting thoughts and memories.

How Is PS Made?

All PS sold today as a dietary supplement is produced from soybeans. This, however, has not always been the case. Originally, PS was extracted from the brains of cows. Because of the possible danger of contamination by "mad cow" disease, PS is now manufactured from soybeans instead. This point is important to mention because virtually all the scientific studies of PS were performed using the product that was made from cow brains, not from soy. Today, however, the only PS available for study and consumption is derived from soy.

PS plays an important role in the transmission of thoughts and memories.

Does it make a difference, you may wonder? Small though it may be, *there is a real chemical difference between the two products.* Although many experts feel that they are so similar they should function identically, it is certainly possible that studies using soy-based PS rather than PS extracted from cow brains would yield different results. The question of how well the soy-derived PS works will only be answered with certainty when new studies are published using it instead of the older form.

What Is the Scientific Evidence for Phosphatidylserine?

Scientists have conducted a considerable amount of research into the effectiveness of PS for Alzheimer's disease and non-Alzheimer's dementia. A total of over 1,000 people have participated in double-blind studies, and

Harold's Story

Harold was an 84-year-old former professional golfer in the very early stages of Alzheimer's disease. He was willing to face the fact bravely, but he wanted to avail himself of any treatment that might extend the time he could participate actively in life. He had tried the medication tacrine, which seemed to help, but he developed a bad reaction to it almost immediately. Next he tried ginkgo, but after 6 weeks neither he nor his wife had noticed any improvement. He came to me wondering whether I knew any other options he might try.

After hearing his story I suggested that he try either phosphatidylserine or L-acetylcarnitine (described in the next chapter). I explained to him that these supplements almost certainly worked differently from ginkgo, and were worth a try. He decided to try phosphatidylserine first. As might be expected from the results of the scientific studies described in this chapter, within 4 weeks Harold's memory and mental function had clearly improved.

—Steven Bratman, M.D.

taken together the evidence strongly suggests that PS is indeed an effective treatment for severe memory loss and mental impairment.

The largest of these double-blind studies enrolled 494 individuals with significant mental impairment.[1] Over a period of 6 months, they were given either placebo or 300 mg of PS daily. As compared to the placebo group, participants taking PS showed significantly greater improvements in memory and mental function. The benefit was roughly comparable to what we have seen with studies involving ginkgo. Improvements were also noticed in mood and behavior of the participants.

Other double-blind studies involving a total of over 500 participants have also shown positive results in treating Alzheimer's and non-Alzheimer's dementia.[2–9]

Just as with ginkgo, there is no solid evidence that PS can help people with ordinary age-related memory loss. However, because it appears to be effective for more than one type of dementia, it certainly seems logical to guess that it might have a general memory-enhancing effect.

How Does PS Work?

We do not know how PS works to improve mental function, but scientists have advanced a few

Double-blind studies involving a total of about 1,000 people strongly suggest that PS is indeed an effective treatment for severe memory loss and mental impairment.

different theories. One of the most popular suggests that PS improves the integrity of our brain cells.

As we get older, free radicals can damage the membranes of all cells, including neurons. In the brain, these membranes are necessary for proper transmission of the electrical and chemical messages that carry our thoughts and memories. Since PS composes a significant part of these membranes, some researchers theorize that taking PS as a dietary supplement helps provides "fresh" PS for "rejuvenating" these damaged membranes. This could improve memory and mental function. However, this theory is pretty speculative, and no direct evidence supports it.

Another theory involves the immune system. Certain immune cells called *phagocytes* have the capacity to re-move cells that are aged or damaged. They seem to be attracted to PS.[10] Normally, PS is found on the *inside* of the membranes of brain cells. As these cells get old and ready to die, PS is transported to the *outside* of the cell membranes. It has been suggested that PS may act as a "flag" to signal the immune system that certain brain cells are ready for destruction,[11,12] something like the red flag on our mailboxes that lets the postman know there's mail to be picked up.

How PS works is not yet known.

According to this theory, when you take PS supplements, it serves as a "decoy" for the white blood cells. They run around devouring the extra PS in the bloodstream and thus are too busy to attack brain cells. However, this theory has several flaws, not the least of which is the fact that aged and damaged brain cells probably need to be devoured anyway.

Other theories involve the possible effects of PS on brain chemistry. For example, according to one animal study, PS appears to boost brain levels of acetylcholine.[13,14] You may remember from earlier in the book that acetylcholine plays a critical role in the transmission of nerve impulses, and that in people with Alzheimer's disease the level of acetylcholine in the brain is reduced. The drug tacrine (discussed in chapter 10) works by raising acetylcholine levels. PS may do the same.

None of these theories is proven, but it is safe to say this: PS probably doesn't work in the same way that ginkgo works. This means that one treatment might be helpful if the other isn't (see previous sidebar, Harold's Story).

Dosage

PS is usually taken in doses of 100 mg 2 to 3 times daily. After maximum effect is achieved, the dose can sometimes be reduced to 100 mg daily without losing benefit. It is not necessary to take PS with food.

Safety Issues

PS is generally regarded as safe. Side effects are rare and appear to be limited to mild digestive distress, such as nausea or minor stomachache. However, formal toxicity studies have not been performed.

There is one theoretical risk with PS, related to the immune theory of how it might work. As I described above, PS on the outside of a cell membrane appears to act as a red flag to indicate that the cell needs to be destroyed. According to this theory, supplemental PS acts as a decoy and prevents the destruction of "flagged" brain cells. However, there is some concern among scientists that long-term use of supplemental PS might protect the wrong cells as well—specifically, cancer cells that really need to be destroyed. Long-term studies are necessary to properly evaluate this concern.

Is PS Safe During Pregnancy and While Nursing?

Researchers have not yet conducted tests or studies on the use of PS by pregnant or nursing mothers. Considering this lack of information, it's best to avoid using it during pregnancy, while trying to get pregnant, or while nursing.

Is PS Safe for Children?

Just as there's no reason children would need to take ginkgo, there's also no reason why children should take PS.

Is PS Safe for Those with Liver or Kidney Disease?

People with liver or kidney disease have to exercise partic-

PS is generally regarded as safe.

ular caution in using drugs of any kind. Natural products are no exception. If you or your loved one has a disease or disorder of the kidneys or liver, it is important that you consult with your family physician before using PS.

Drug Interactions

Medical practitioners are concerned that PS, like ginkgo, may have a blood-thinning effect.[15] For this reason, if you are taking a blood-thinning or anti-coagulant medication such as warfarin (Coumadin), heparin, aspirin, or pentoxifylline (Trental), consult your medical doctor before you take PS. It is also at least conceivable that PS could interact with other natural products that have a mild blood-thinning effect, such as garlic, ginkgo, and high dose vitamin E supplements.

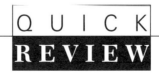

QUICK REVIEW

- PS is an essential component in the membranes of cells, including brain cells.
- Double-blind studies enrolling about 1,000 people have found that PS is an effective treatment for severe age-related memory loss, such as Alzheimer's disease.

- There is no good evidence as yet that PS can help people with ordinary age-related memory loss, but as with ginkgo, it seems logical to guess that it might.

- The suggested dosage of PS is 100 mg 2 or 3 times a day. Once good results develop, you can try reducing your dose to 100 mg daily to see if it still works.

- We don't know how PS actually works. However, several theories have been suggested. One theory suggests that it improves the integrity of our brain cells. Another theory involves PS acting as a "decoy" to prevent premature destruction of aging brain cells. Yet another possible explanation suggests that PS improves brain function by boosting brain levels of acetylcholine.

- PS is generally regarded as safe. However, if you are taking any blood-thinning or anti-coagulant herbs, supplements, or medications, consult with your physician before you take PS.

Other Natural Treatments to Improve Memory

E vidence suggests that several other natural treatments besides ginkgo can improve memory and mental functioning. (Actually, as I'll explain, some aren't exactly "natural.") This chapter will tell you about the most promising of these supplements.

Again, we have the same situation we found with ginkgo and PS—because it's easier to get funding for studies of a disease, almost all the research has concerned severe conditions such as Alzheimer's disease and multi-infarct dementia.

L-acetylcarnitine: May Imitate Acetylcholine

L-acetylcarnitine (el-uh-SEE-tuhl-car-nah-teen) is a special form of a nutrient called "L-carnitine" found in meat. In the body, L-carnitine plays a major role in "burning" fat to make energy. L-carnitine is widely used as a natural treatment for heart disease, but the slightly modified form

L-acetylcarnitine appears to be helpful for conditions involving memory and mental functioning.

Theories on How L-acetylcarnitine Works

We're not entirely sure how L-acetylcarnitine works. One major theory holds that it functions by imitating the function of the substance acetylcholine. As you may recall from chapter 3, acetylcholine plays a major role in the brain. In people with Alzheimer's disease, acetylcholine production appears to be impaired. L-acetylcarnitine, according to this theory, partially makes up for a deficiency in this important brain chemical.

According to the leading theory, L-acetylcarnitine works by imitating the important neurotransmitter acetylcholine.

While there are other theories about how it works,[1,2] we do know at least that L-acetylcarnitine easily crosses over from the blood into the brain. This means that the L-acetylcarnitine you swallow in a tablet can directly affect your brain chemistry.[3]

What Is the Scientific Evidence for L-acetylcarnitine?

L-acetylcarnitine is one of the best-studied natural treatments for memory and mental functioning. Researchers have enrolled a total of over 1,000 participants in double-blind placebo-controlled studies on the use of L-acetylcarnitine for Alzheimer's disease and non-Alzheimer's dementia.[4-13] Most of this research had at least slightly positive results.

For example, one double-blind trial followed 130 individuals with mild to moderate Alzheimer's disease for

Lou's Story

One patient I see, a 72-year-old man with severe mental impairment, has had a lifelong dislike of synthetic medications. This feeling does not seem to have grown out of bad experiences. Rather, it seems to be part of his philosophy of life.

Respecting his predilections, which she knew well, his wife had tried treating Lou with ginkgo. Unfortunately, it didn't help. She then tried to get him to take the drug tacrine (see chapter 10). However, although it seemed to be effective, she had to fight with him constantly to get him to take it.

She then began to search the Internet and discovered L-acetylcarnitine. She asked me whether it was worth a try. I

---

1 year.[14] All participants worsened over that time, but according to 14 different measurements of mental function and behavior, the treated group deteriorated more slowly. However, the difference was not very large, and it was only statistically significant for a few of the rating scales used.

Another double-blind trial of over 500 individuals also found evidence that L-acetylcarnitine can slow the progression of Alzheimer's disease and non-Alzheimer's dementia.[15] Furthermore, benefits were seen in placebo-controlled (but not double-blind) studies involving a total of over 700 additional participants.[16, 17]

Some studies, however, have not found any benefit. In particular, a recent year-long double-blind placebo-controlled trial enrolling 431 participants found no significant improvement in the L-acetylcarnitine treated group at all.[18]

said it might be because this substance is thought to work somewhat similarly to tacrine.

After about 4 weeks at a dose of 500 mg three times per day, Lou seemed to improve. His wife said that he was much easier to talk to and took care of himself more predictably. Because L-acetylcarnitine wasn't a "drug," he was happy to take it.

Was this a true benefit or wishful thinking? I don't know. As described in this chapter, the research evidence for L-acetylcarnitine is somewhat contradictory. We don't have as solid evidence for its effectiveness as we do for ginkgo and phosphatidylserine.

—Steven Bratman, M.D.

The most likely explanation for the negative outcome in this well-designed study is that L-acetylcarnitine produces only a small benefit at most. Still, since it apparently works by a completely different mechanism than ginkgo, you might find it worth a try if the herb does not work for you.

Dosage

The typical dose of L-acetylcarnitine is 500 mg to 1,000 mg 3 times a day. Unfortunately, this is a very expensive supplement, easily costing more than $80 per month.

Safety Issues

L-acetylcarnitine seems to be a very safe supplement, consistent with the fact that carnitine itself is present widely in the body. The maximum safe dose is not known for young children, pregnant or nursing women, or those with liver or kidney problems.

Huperzine A:
Works Like the Standard Drug Tacrine

Huperzine A (HUP-er-zeen) is an extremely potent chemical derived from a particular type of club moss (*Huperzia serrata* [Thumb] Trev.). Like caffeine and cocaine, huperzine A is a medicinally active, plant-derived chemical that belongs to the class known as *alkaloids*. It was first isolated in 1948 by Chinese scientists.[19]

Huperzine A inhibits the enzyme *acetylcholinesterase* (uh-SEE-tul-co-lin-ES-ter-ase). This enzyme breaks down acetylcholine, which as we saw in chapter 2 seems to play an important role in mental function. When the enzyme that breaks it down is inhibited, acetylcholine levels in the brain tend to rise. As we'll see in chapter 10, drugs that inhibit acetylcholinesterase (such as tacrine and donepezil) seem to improve memory and mental functioning in people with Alzheimer's and other severe conditions. The research on huperzine A indicates that it works in much the same way.

Huperzine A works very much like the drugs tacrine and donepezil, but even more specifically.

The chemical action of huperzine A is very precise and specific. It "fits" into a niche on the enzyme where acetylcholine is supposed to attach.[20,21] Because huperzine A is in the way, the enzyme can't grab and destroy acetylcholine. This mechanism has been demonstrated by considerable scientific work, including sophisticated computer modeling of the shape of the molecule.[22]

Although it originally comes from a plant, huperzine A is highly purified in a laboratory and is just a single chemical. It is just not much like an herb. Herbs contain hundreds or thousands of chemicals. In this way, huperzine A resembles drugs such as digoxin, codeine, Sudafed, and vincristine (a chemotherapy drug), which are also highly purified chemicals taken from plants. If we wish to call huperzine A a natural treatment, we need to call these (and dozens of other standard drugs) natural as well.

This naturally occurring chemical is quite powerful and should be considered more drug-like than herb-like in its actions. Dietary supplements such as L-acetylcarnitine and vitamin C are also single chemicals, but since they are ordinarily found in the diet and in the body, calling them "natural treatments" is reasonable. But few people eat the huperzia club moss for dinner as a source of huperzine A.

Huperzine A should probably be subjected to the rigorous controls that apply to other drugs. However, for complex reasons, this is impractical, and it is being sold as a dietary supplement in the United States. In my opinion, this is unfortunate.

What Is the Scientific Evidence for Huperzine A?

Many experiments have found that huperzine A can improve memory skills in aged animals as well as in younger animals whose memories have been deliberately impaired.[23–38]

Some of the best research on humans so far was done in a clinical trial involving 103 people with Alzheimer's disease. Participants in this placebo-controlled study were given either huperzine A or a placebo twice a day for 8 weeks. About 60% of the treated participants showed improvements in memory, thinking, and behavioral functions

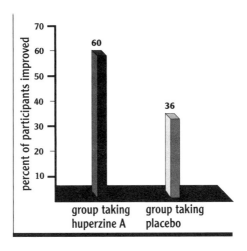

Figure 8. *Double-blind study shows that huperzine A improved memory, thinking, and behavioral functions* (Xu et al., 1995)

compared to 36% of the placebo-treated group (see figure 8). No severe side effects were reported, and the authors concluded that huperzine A is a promising drug for symptomatic treatment of Alzheimer's disease.[39]

Dosage
Although huperzine A is sold as a dietary supplement, it should not be confused with an ordinary herb. This substance is a highly potent compound with a recommended dose of only 50 mcg (0.05 mg) twice a day for age-related memory loss. I recommend using it only under a doctor's supervision.

Safety Issues
Perhaps because it works so specifically, huperzine A appears to have few side effects. However, children, pregnant

Not Your Average "Dietary Supplement"

Legally classified as a "dietary supplement" and available over the counter in the United States, vinpocetine has been advertised as a "better than ginkgo" treatment that can improve memory even in younger people. However, European physicians consulted during the writing of this book were surprised to hear that vinpocetine was considered a "dietary supplement" or herbal treatment in the United States. In Europe it is considered a standard synthetic drug. Although it might indeed be a promising treatment for memory loss, in my opinion it should go through the standard drug-approval process and be regulated like other prescription drugs.

or nursing women, or those with high blood pressure or severe liver or kidney disease should not take huperzine A except on a doctor's recommendation. We also don't know whether huperzine A interacts adversely with any drugs.

Vinpocetine: Clearly Not a Natural Treatment

Vinpocetine (vin-PO-se-teen) is another "dietary supplement" that is actually more like a drug than an herb, perhaps even more so than huperzine A. It is a chemical derived from vincamine, a constituent found in the leaves of common periwinkle (*Vinca minor* L.). A different periwinkle, the Madagascaran periwinkle (*Catharanthus roseus* G. Don.), is the source of the anti-cancer drugs vincristine and vinblastine.

Developed in Hungary over 20 years ago, vinpocetine is sold in Europe as a drug under the name Cavinton. In the United States it is available as a "dietary supplement," although the substance probably doesn't fit that category by any rational definition. Unlike huperzine A, vinpocetine doesn't occur in nature at all. Producing it requires significant chemical work performed in the laboratory. Chemists start with a substance found in the seeds of various African plants (they use this source instead of periwinkle for economic reasons), and then use various chemical processes to transform it into vinpocetine.[40]

We don't know how vinpocetine works, although there are numerous theories. There is some evidence that vinpocetine can safeguard brain cells against damage caused by lack of oxygen.[41] However, whether this effect really has anything to do with its effects on mental function remains unclear.

What Is the Scientific Evidence for Vinpocetine?

A significant level of evidence supports the idea that vinpocetine can enhance memory and mental function. However, most of the studies that have been reported predate the modern understanding of Alzheimer's disease and rely on the outmoded concept that dementia is caused by a chronically marginal oxygen supply to the brain.

One 3-month double-blind placebo-controlled study followed 84 individuals with age-related mental impairment.[42] According to several standard rating scales, the severity of the illness improved by a statistically significant margin in the treatment group as compared to the placebo group. Similarly positive results have been seen in many other studies,[43] although at least one study did not find benefit.[44]

Dosage

Vinpocetine is available in 10 mg capsules, usually taken 3 times per day. This supplement is probably best taken with meals, as it is better absorbed that way.[45] I recommend that it only be used on physician advice.

Rosemary for Remembrance?

In Shakespeare's play *Hamlet,* the distraught Ophelia carries a bouquet of herbs including rosemary, which she says is "for remembrance." As this allusion suggests, rosemary is a traditional folk treatment used to sharpen memory. Unfortunately, no real evidence is available to support using rosemary to treat memory loss.

Safety Issues

No serious side effects have been reported in any of the clinical trials. However, like ginkgo, vinpocetine should not be combined with blood-thinning drugs such as Coumadin (warfarin), heparin, aspirin, or Trental (pentoxifylline) except on the advice of a physician.[46] Vinpocetine might also interact with natural substances that thin the blood as well, including ginkgo, phosphatidylserine (PS), garlic, and high dose vitamin E. Safety in pregnant women or those with severe liver or kidney disease has not been established.

One study found that ginseng improved reaction time and abstract thinking; it did *not* improve memory or the ability to concentrate.

Other Herbs

Now we return to the world of real herbs, as opposed to the highly synthesized and purified herbal derivatives we've just discussed. Among commonly available herbs, both rosemary and the Chinese herb ginseng have a traditional reputation for enhancing memory. While little evidence supports the theory that rosemary is effective, at least some scientific evidence supports the use of ginseng.

Many books have been written on ginseng—both the Asian and American species (which are true ginsengs) and so-called Siberian ginseng (which is not a true ginseng).

One double-blind study evaluated the effects of Asian ginseng on mental function in 112 healthy middle-aged adults.[47] Participants received either placebo or 400 mg daily of a standardized ginseng extract daily for 8 to 9 weeks. Significant improvements in abstract thinking ability were seen in the treated group, whereas the placebo group did not show improvement. Interestingly, ginseng did *not* appear to help memory or concentration. If this benefit is confirmed by other studies, ginseng may prove to be a complement to ginkgo for enhancing mental function.

Ginseng appears to be quite a safe herb. For more information on how to use it and what safety considerations to keep in mind, see *The Natural Pharmacist: Your Complete Guide to Herbs.*

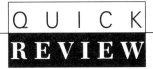

QUICK REVIEW

- L-acetylcarnitine is a derivative of a substance found in meat. Although the scientific record is mixed, overall the results suggest that L-acetylcarnitine can slightly improve memory and mental function in those with Alzheimer's and non-Alzheimer's dementia.

- Huperzine A is an extremely potent chemical isolated from a species of club moss. This compound specifically inhibits the enzyme that metabolizes acetylcholine, thereby raising acetylcholine levels. This is the same mechanism of action as other drugs already approved for treating loss of mental function.

- Although it's legally classified as a "dietary supplement," in many ways huperzine A is more like a drug than an herb.

- Vinpocetine is a synthetic chemical that also should be classified as a drug rather than a dietary supplement. It has been available as the drug Cavinton in Europe for about 20 years. Vinpocetine appears to improve memory and mental function.

- The herb ginseng may improve some aspects of thinking ability but does not appear to improve memory.

CHAPTER

TEN

Conventional Treatments for Alzheimer's Disease

I n previous chapters, we've discussed several natural treatments that might be of help with mild or serious memory loss. There are no approved prescription medications available for mild memory loss, but several medications have been approved for treating symptoms of Alzheimer's disease. This chapter describes the leading conventional medications, as well as other medical therapies used to treat severe mental impairment.

Sometimes healthy people who are worried about normal age-related memory loss ask their doctor for one of these prescription medications. Doctors are usually reluctant to comply, for good reason. Not only is there no evidence that these medications can help a healthy person (that is, a person who is not suffering from Alzheimer's disease), but these drugs cause various troublesome side effects.

As we've seen, there isn't much evidence to show that ginkgo works for healthy people, either. However, ginkgo is almost free of side effects, so there is less risk in trying it.

Cholinesterase Inhibitors: May Reduce Symptoms of Alzheimer's Disease

Two drugs are currently available in the United States that can temporarily improve memory and mental functioning in people with Alzheimer's disease. Tacrine (Cognex) and donepezil (Aricept) both increase the level of acetylcholine in the brain.

As we saw in chapter 3, acetylcholine is an important neurotransmitter—that is, a chemical that carries impulses between nerve cells in the brain. Since people with Alzheimer's disease have reduced levels of acetylcholine in their brains, scientists have speculated that raising the level of acetylcholine might improve symptoms of Alzheimer's disease.

Acetylcholine is constantly produced and just as constantly destroyed. One way to raise acetylcholine levels is to inhibit one side of this process— prevent it from being broken down. Normally, acetylcholine is deactivated by enzymes called

Tacrine (Cognex) produces significant benefits in about 30% of people with Alzheimer's disease who take it.

cholinesterases. The two approved Alzheimer's medications, tacrine and donepezil (as well as huperzine A, which was discussed in chapter 9), inhibit these enzymes. The net result is that acetylcholine levels rise.

However, cholinesterase inhibitors can affect the stomach, which makes them risky for individuals already at risk for developing ulcers. This includes those who are taking common nonsteroidal anti-inflammatory drugs (NSAIDs) such as

Treatments for Alzheimer's Disease: Prevention Versus Symptom Reduction

As we saw in chapter 3, Alzheimer's disease is caused by a progressive death of nerve cells in the brain. As yet, no cure exists for this condition. However, medications such as tacrine and donepezil can relieve the symptoms of Alzheimer's disease and help those who have the condition function at an improved level. But these medications don't actually prevent nerve cells from dying or even slow the rate at which they die.

At present, most researchers think that the cell death in Alzheimer's disease is caused by free radicals—dangerous chemicals in the body that also accelerate heart disease and cancer. The search is on for preventive treatments that could actually protect brain cells from free radicals and thus slow or

aspirin and ibuprofen. There are, however, good reasons why one might be tempted to combine these treatments. As we will see, regular use of certain NSAIDs may help protect brain cells against Alzheimer's disease. But because of the risks, definitely consult your physician before you take both a cholinesterase inhibitor and an NSAID at the same time.

Both tacrine and donepezil are expensive: A 30-day supply costs well over $100.

Tacrine: Reduces Symptoms But Can Irritate the Liver

Tacrine (Cognex) was the first prescription cholinesterase inhibitor to be clinically tested and approved by the FDA even halt the progress of Alzheimer's disease. Antioxidants such as the drug selegiline and vitamin E fight free radicals and may therefore be helpful.

Interestingly, there is some evidence that a group of medications currently in use for completely different problems can both relieve symptoms of Alzheimer's disease as well as slow its progression. These are the nonsteroidal anti-inflammatory drugs, or NSAIDs, used widely to reduce pain, fever, and inflammation. Ibuprofen is one of the most famous of the NSAID drugs. Evidence suggests that these medications can also inhibit certain free radicals that play a role in Alzheimer's disease.

(in 1993). It appears to produce significant benefits in only about 30% of people who try it, but studies have found it significantly more effective than placebo. When tacrine is successful, it improves short-term memory and overall mental functioning.

For example, Ellen was an 84-year-old woman with early symptoms of Alzheimer's disease. A writer by trade, she successfully fought to keep control by keeping careful notes and reminders to herself. This worked for about 6 months; but then her mind began to deteriorate too much. Just at that time, tacrine came on the market. After taking it for a month, Ellen came out from under the shadow of the disease and managed to cope successfully for an additional 6 months. It didn't last forever, but her family is very grateful for that extra time.

Tacrine can cause a variety of side effects including nausea, diarrhea, insomnia, vomiting, muscle cramps, fatigue, and loss of appetite. These are often mild and fade away while the individual is still on treatment. A more serious potential problem is liver inflammation, which occurs in as many as 30 to 50% of those who take tacrine and may require stopping the medication.

In addition, tacrine must be taken four times a day. This annoying dosage schedule should be corrected soon by the approval of a slow-release form of the drug.

Donepezil: Much Like Tacrine, but Safer and Easier to Use

Donepezil (Aricept) was approved for treatment of mild to moderate dementia of the Alzheimer's type in 1996. It works by the same mechanism as tacrine but lasts longer in the body so that you don't need to take it so many times a day. Also, it doesn't appear to irritate the liver. Otherwise it is rather similar. Minor side effects are similar to those seen with tacrine.

On the Horizon: "Second-Generation" Cholinesterase Inhibitors

"Second-generation" cholinesterase inhibitors in development include ENA 713, eptastigmine, and metrifonate.[1] Each has been clinically tested and may be approved soon. These second-generation medications may be superior in various ways to existing drugs, but research has not yet been completed.

Pharmaceutical companies are also currently developing two natural compounds that inhibit cholinesterase as possible treatments for Alzheimer's disease. One of these compounds, physostigmine, is also used for other purposes, such as the treatment of glaucoma and as an antidote to drugs that reduce acetylcholine levels.

Physostigmine is found in the seed of the Calabar bean, which is also known as the "ordeal bean." The species name of this bean, *venenosum,* means "full of poison." The Calabar bean was used in pre-colonial Africa by a secret society of the Efik tribal people of Nigeria called the Egbo. The Egbo wielded power partly through judicious use of physostigmine.

Donepezil (Aricept) works much like tacrine, but you don't have to take as many pills a day, and it doesn't seem to irritate the liver.

Michael Balick and Paul Cox, in their book *Plants, People, and Culture,* report that a serious offense against the Egbo could result in trial by the ordeal bean of Calabar. William Daniell, a British medical officer stationed in Calabar in 1846, wrote that a person thought to be guilty of witchcraft was forced to swallow a liquid made from these toxic seeds and ordered to walk around until the effects could be felt. If, after a certain period of time, the accused had not succumbed to the poison and died, she was considered proven innocent and set free.

The other natural compound that researchers are currently studying as a possible treatment for Alzheimer's disease is galanthamine from the Caucasian snowdrop plant. Like the Calabar bean, the Caucasian snowdrop inhibits cholinesterase activity.[2]

Finally, as discussed in the last chapter, huperzine A is a specific inhibitor of acetylcholinesterase. But instead of pursuing the drug route, manufacturers have presented it as a dietary supplement.

NSAIDs: May Both Prevent and Treat Alzheimer's Disease

"Nonsteroidal anti-inflammatory drugs" (NSAIDs) is a fancy way of describing medications such as aspirin and ibuprofen (Motrin, Advil, and Nuprin), as well as others

that are available only with a prescription. It's easy to forget that even common, over-the-counter medicines are powerful. But they are. NSAIDs appear to reduce the symptoms of Alzheimer's disease and perhaps slow its progression and even help prevent it. NSAIDs may also help multi-infarct dementia, although this has not been proven.

NSAIDs such as ibuprofen appear to improve the mental functioning of people with Alzheimer's disease by relieving inflammation of the brain tissue.

In Alzheimer's disease, the tangles and plaques that form in the brain lead to inflammation of the brain tissue. This inflammation not only impairs brain function, it also produces free radicals that injure brain cells. It seems reasonable that anti-inflammatory drugs might help relieve symptoms as well as protect brain cells from further injury.

A 1993 study found that mental functioning improved slightly in people with Alzheimer's disease who were given the NSAID indomethacin, while it declined in those on placebo.[3] In a later review of 210 people with Alzheimer's disease, those who took NSAIDs did better and declined less quickly than those who were not taking these drugs.[4] Other research has also tended to support the idea that NSAIDs can provide protection against Alzheimer's disease.[5]

However, it's not yet clear that a healthy person with a family history of Alzheimer's disease could reduce the risk of developing it by taking NSAIDs. More research is needed, especially since long-term use of NSAIDs involves definite health risks, primarily harm to the digestive tract.

The NSAIDs for which there is some evidence of a helpful effect in Alzheimer's disease include ibuprofen (Motrin, Advil, Nuprin), indomethacin (Indocin), meclofenamate (Meclomen), naproxen (Naprosyn), and maybe aspirin. However, the evidence is far from solid at this point. Much more work needs to be done before we can say that the benefits outweigh the known risks of these drugs. Do not take NSAIDs on a daily basis without consulting your doctor.

Antioxidants: May Slow the Progression of Alzheimer's Disease

The drug selegiline (Eldepryl) is used to slow the progression of Parkinson's disease. One study of 341 participants suggests that it, as well as vitamin E, may also be helpful in slowing the progression of Alzheimer's disease.[6]

Although we don't know precisely how selegiline works, the medication is known to have antioxidant properties. As I mentioned early, antioxidants fight free radicals, which are thought to play a role in the development of Alzheimer's disease (as well as Parkinson's disease). Vitamin E is also an antioxidant. This study evaluated both treatments, as well as their combination, and compared the results against placebo treatment.

Participants with relatively mild Alzheimer's symptoms received selegiline (10 mg a day), vitamin E (2,000 IU a day), both, or placebo for 2 years. The results showed that both vitamin E and selegiline significantly increased the time before the disease became severe. In other words, they slowed the progression of the disease. Interestingly, selegiline alone was better than the combined treatment.

Slowing the Progression
of Alzheimer's Disease

When David found out he had Alzheimer's disease, it felt like a death sentence. His mind was still active enough to know what was happening to him. Furthermore, when he started taking donepezil, his mind "cleared" substantially, and he really knew what lay ahead. He was a single man with no close relatives, and he began to view the nursing home as a fugitive might once have viewed the hangman's noose.

Struggling against the limitations of his failing mind, David researched on the Internet and found out that the drug selegiline appeared to be effective at slowing the progression of Alz-

---

If other studies corroborate these results, either selegiline or vitamin E may become standard treatments for Alzheimer's disease. Keep in mind that 2,000 IU of vitamin E is a very high dose that should not be taken except under physician supervision. Like so many other natural treatments used for Alzheimer's disease, high dose vitamin E "thins" the blood and may present a risk of bleeding complications. I would especially recommend medical advice before combining it with blood-thinning drugs such as warfarin (Coumadin), heparin, pentoxifylline (Trental), and aspirin. High dose vitamin E might also conceivably interact

Two large clinical trials are currently looking into the benefits of estrogen therapy for Alzheimer's disease.

heimer's disease. He ordered a copy of the study on which this idea was based and brought it in to his physician. Without any hesitation, the doctor prescribed it for him. "What do you have to lose?" he said.

David is still independent, a year later, and is writing his memoirs. How much of this is due to the selegiline, no one can say. But he's grateful for the opportunity to stay in control of his life a little longer. I look forward to reading what he is writing—he had an interesting life, and it isn't over yet.

with natural substances that mildly thin the blood, such as ginkgo, phosphatidylserine, and garlic.

Estrogen Therapy: May Prevent Alzheimer's Disease, but We Need More Evidence

Preliminary evidence suggests that the hormone estrogen exerts a protective effect against Alzheimer's disease, at least in women. Estrogen is naturally produced in the body, and though men's bodies do produce small amounts of it, estrogen is primarily a female hormone.

Estrogen plays a major role in a woman's reproductive cycle. During menopause, a woman's estrogen level declines as she ceases to ovulate. Because estrogen does a number of good things for the body, such as protecting the heart and bones, many women take supplemental estrogen after menopause.

Alzheimer's and the Art of Communication

Richard was a man in his 80s who had begun to exhibit classic signs of Alzheimer's disease. His memory of events and common knowledge was clearly failing. He became easily lost and disoriented. He could no longer drive safely. As his capabilities diminished, he became increasingly irritable and prone to frustration. His family recognized these signs and began to prepare for him to move into a managed care facility in their state. Fearing resistance, they were wise enough not to insist but to suggest. They asked, "Did you ever think of coming back to Kansas when you can't handle things any longer?"

Richard replied, "Yes, I'd like that." When they tentatively described the nursing home they had in mind, he actually thanked them for the information. His family was relieved and

Recent headlines in major media have trumpeted the possibility that estrogen use can reduce the incidence of Alzheimer's disease. However, the evidence is not yet strong. While some investigations have suggested that estrogen protects women against Alzheimer's disease,[7–10] all the studies published thus far have serious flaws.[11,12] The evidence is not anywhere near as solid as the media has made it sound.

Currently this question is being studied in two large and properly designed clinical trials: the Women's Health Initiative and the Heart and Estrogen Replacement Therapy Study. The results of these two major studies should help provide some definitive answers regarding the effectiveness of long-term estrogen therapy for Alzheimer's disease and other conditions, as well its potential risks.[13] The results, however, will not be available for years.

more than a bit surprised. Richard had always been a strong-willed man—he was a former Marine and a World War II veteran—but he seemed to grasp what was happening to him. More important, the family had managed to communicate their concern without offending him. Had they tried to order him around, they would have likely gotten a different answer.

Communicating with a loved one with a severe mental impairment is one of the most stressful tasks a family can face. Some families, like Richard's, are able to cope successfully, but not all afflicted people are able to respond as well as Richard did to his family's concern. Counseling is one approach that can help families learn new strategies for communicating with each other in the face of a member's severe mental impairment.

In the meantime, I don't suggest taking estrogen simply in hopes that it will prevent Alzheimer's disease. If you want to take it to prevent osteoporosis or heart disease, that's fine. But considering how weak current evidence is for an estrogen–Alzheimer's disease link, taking it for this reason alone probably isn't advisable. There are very real fears that estrogen replacement therapy can significantly increase your risk of developing breast cancer, and if it is not combined with a progestin, it definitely increases the risk of uterine cancer.

We're not sure exactly how estrogen might protect against Alzheimer's disease. Estrogen improves blood flow to the brain, boosts acetylcholine production, may help prevent the formation of plaque, and is an antioxidant.[14] Any and all of these effects might play a role in its proposed anti Alzheimer's activity.

Hydergine: An Older Drug Seldom Used Today

A combination drug named hydergine has been used for the treatment of impaired mental function in the elderly. A review of the scientific literature shows that it might provide some modest benefit, but more research is needed to firmly establish whether this is actually so.[15] A chemical modification of ergot alkaloids (drugs usually used for migraine headaches), hydergine is seldom prescribed today.

Psychotherapy and Other Nondrug Approaches to Alzheimer's Disease

Drugs aren't the only possible approach to Alzheimer's disease. In conventional medicine, psychotherapy is sometimes recommended as a helpful treatment in the early stages of the disease. In addition to memory loss, dementia brings disturbing changes in personality. These changes can be as distressing to the person with Alzheimer's and to the caregivers as is the decline in memory. A once-cheerful relative with Alzheimer's may slowly become demanding, difficult, unreasonable, or even aggressive. It's not clear what causes these symptoms, but it is certainly natural that a person with increasing mental impairment would feel frustrated, depressed, and angry.

In the early stages of Alzheimer's disease, psychotherapy or counseling can help ease the frustration and the other troubling emotional or behavioral changes. Practical, outcome-oriented therapy can teach both the person with Alzheimer's disease and his or her caregivers useful strategies for managing potentially stressful everyday tasks, such as bathing and eating. One way to deal with a severely afflicted person's level of emotional stress is to avoid situations that provoke frustration. A psychotherapist or counselor who specializes in severe age-related mental impairment can help explain the afflicted person's emotional needs to caregivers, and suggest practical strategies for avoiding stress.

Another type of therapy aims to bolster the cognitive functioning of those with Alzheimer's by teaching them basic life skills and information. For example, classes that specifically teach people with Alzheimer's how to manage their disease may help them through the first part of the condition. Some people with early Alzheimer's can compensate for the loss of their mental faculties by careful use of lists and reminders. Clearly, however, such techniques don't address the root causes of severe mental impairment, and mental function will eventually decline so much that these memory aids are no longer useful. Furthermore, this method may increase the frustration of people with Alzheimer's who feel as if they are being made to walk in spite of a broken leg.

Yet another psychological approach is to stimulate mental functioning through the use of mild, enjoyable exercises or activities. This might be called the "use it or lose it" school of therapy, and we can all benefit from this approach. For a person with Alzheimer's disease or multi-infarct dementia, even stroking a cat or taking a walk can be a beneficial, stimulating experience. If nothing else, enjoyable movement can help improve an afflicted person's mood. However, the benefits of this kind of therapy for severe mental impairment also seem to be short-lived.

Finally, for mildly affected people, emotion-oriented counseling can help with the difficult adjustment to life with a severe mental impairment. Caregivers, too, may find counseling helpful in dealing with the significant emotional stress of caring for a severely affected loved one.

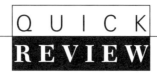

QUICK REVIEW

- No prescription medications are available to treat ordinary age-related memory loss, but some conventional treatments—both psychotherapy and medication—can help with Alzheimer's disease.

- Among drug treatments, the cholinesterase inhibitors tacrine (Cognex) and donepezil (Aricept) appear to offer the most benefit at present. More drugs in this class are currently under development including the longer-acting inhibitors eptastigmine and metrifonate, as well as the natural products physostigmine and galanthamine. These medications don't reverse or prevent Alzheimer's disease, but they can improve mental functioning in the short term.

- Tacrine and donepezil are effective in about 30% of people with Alzheimer's disease who try these medications. However, tacrine can cause liver inflammation, and it must be taken in 4 doses a day.

- Nonsteroidal anti-inflammatory drugs (NSAIDs) may reduce symptoms of Alzheimer's disease and also possibly slow its progression. Regular use of NSAIDs has also been associated with a lower overall incidence of Alzheimer's disease. However, because these medications offer significant risks, they should not be taken on a daily basis except on the advice of a physician.

- Antioxidant substances such as selegiline and vitamin E appear to help slow the progression of Alzheimer's disease.

- Weak evidence suggests that regular use of estrogen reduces the chance of developing Alzheimer's disease.

- Psychotherapy may also offer some help to people suffering from dementia, as well as their families.

Other Ways to Sharpen Memory

T om often complains about his memory. "My memory used to be so good that I couldn't remember the last time I forgot anything. Now it's so bad, I can't remember the last time I forgot something! I meet someone and can't connect a name with the face. I go to the store and return home with only half of what I need. Every morning, I spend 5 minutes looking for my car keys. It's terrible."

Memory is as integral a part of life as is eating and breathing. Only when you start to have memory lapses do you begin to appreciate what we all tend to take for granted. Our memory ties pieces of our lives together. It allows us to make both the necessary connections for daily functioning and those needed to fully appreciate the things that bring us joy. Are there ways to improve your memory? (And if there are, why didn't they teach them in school?) Are there things you can do to compensate for a poor or failing memory?

It is often said that the mind is just another muscle that can be strengthened with exercise. While a bit of an oversimplification, there is some truth to it. With *good training,* you can improve mental functions.

From physical aids to special techniques, you can do many things to cope with or improve a poor memory. Some methods are astounding in their simplicity and effectiveness; others are more complex, requiring learning and practice. Certain techniques are aimed at developing a super memory, enabling recall of impressive numbers of items.

It is possible to sharpen your memory in much the same way as an athlete trains—with a deliberate and organized effort.

Since few people have an interest in memorizing the Periodic Table or the Newark phone directory, this chapter will be concerned with improving your *everyday* memory. Here are tips, hints, and techniques for learning how to better remember people's names, addresses, and phone numbers; where you put your car keys; what you need at the supermarket; and the rest of life's little details.

The Basics of Memory Improvement

Some of what you can do to start on the road to improving your memory is merely a matter of attitude adjustment. Since memory is a thought process, it follows that you can make your memory better by improving your thought processes. Much of it is that simple.

Make a commitment to improving your memory. Once you decide to sharpen your memory or to improve a poor one, you've already taken the first and most important step: commitment. The beginnings of all memory improvement methods start with a decision to make an effort. Try some of the different techniques for improving your memory described in this chapter and see which ones work best for you. Set goals and assess your progress daily. Commit time and energy to this project.

Take a positive attitude.   Stop telling yourself that you have a bad memory. Be positive. Don't think of yourself as absentminded. Expect more from yourself. You'll be surprised how much difference this simple attitude change can make.

Reduce stress.   Stress makes you think less clearly for many reasons, psychological as well as physical. Confusion, frustration, and the hurried pace of life these days all are impediments to a good memory. If you've ever had something "on the tip of your tongue," you'll understand how poorly the memory can work when you're under pressure. Only after you relax does the tidbit of information usually come to mind.

> **The beginnings of all memory improvement methods start with a decision to make an effort.**

Make an effort to keep calm.
If your daily life is especially stressful, consider one of the many stress-reduction techniques available. If you're expecting a stressful situation, try one of the memory aids below, such as notes or reminders.

Focus on what you need to remember.   Simply paying more attention to the things you need to remember can work wonders. Make a conscious effort to "save" memories. When you're parking at the mall, look around before you leave your car to see just where you've parked. Focusing, paying attention, and *making an effort to remember* are the simplest techniques for improving your recall.

Simply paying more attention to the things you need to remember can work wonders.

Repeat the things you need to remember. This is the basis for virtually all study techniques, and it will work wonders in your everyday life. The more you repeat something, the more likely you are to remember it. The more you call a phone number, the less likely it is you'll have to look it up; and the more you see a face, the more likely you'll be able to remember a name to go with it. Driving somewhere with some complicated directions? Go over the directions several times before you leave. If you have something you need to remember, go over it a few times. Making mental pictures works very well for many of us. Visualize what you need to remember. Allow images to come to mind and use them.

Relate the item to yourself; give it meaning. Remembering unassociated facts or items is difficult. Understanding something is *knowing* it, and knowing it is key to making it part of your memory. Details that have meaning to you, that make sense to you, are much more easily remembered than isolated particulars.

Talk to yourself out loud. If you are trying to remember something, say it out loud. Whether it's "Yes, I took my pills today," reading your shopping list out loud, or reminding yourself to stop at the cleaners on the way home, you'll find that verbalizing works to get things into your memory.

What You Can Do to Help Yourself Remember

No one has a perfect memory. Everyone uses tricks from time to time to remind themselves of names or appointments. You can use many techniques for reminding yourself of events, anniversaries, short lists of items, and other details that don't rely on your memory. Some of these are tried-and-true techniques, such as making lists and notes. Other hints may be new to you, such as memorization tricks.

The more you repeat something, the more likely you are to remember it.

The Paper Memory: Making Notes

Notes and lists are the most common memory "extenders." From shopping lists to reminders, the very act of writing things down can help you to remember. Use a date book or calendar to keep track of important appointments. Keep a "Do List" detailing what you need to accomplish and when. Make shopping lists, leave yourself notes, and in general, put down on paper what you want to remember. Don't forget to keep your notes organized and to look at them daily. If you need to, hang your notes where you'll see them—on the refrigerator, the bathroom mirror, even the TV set.

Get Organized!

Arnie lived alone and in total chaos. Things were where he last set them down. It might take him 5 minutes to find a jar of pickles in his refrigerator or 20 minutes to locate his slippers. In such a state of disarray, it was impossible for him to remember where anything was. His life was a puzzle, and he spent most of his time looking for the pieces.

Armed (with a List!) and Ready

Eve was a 72-year-old woman who charged through life taking on all challenges with energy. Since her retirement, she'd volunteered as a Girl Friday at a local animal shelter. Her duties for several years had included answering phones, walking some dogs, and purchasing supplies for the shelter's front office. Lately, however, she was beginning to be bothered by her failing memory, and she felt her memory was affecting her personality and lifestyle. As she told her neighbor, "I used to be able to go to the office supply store, get what I needed, and get back to the shelter in record time. Now, I walk in the store, and I can't remember the first thing I need. Also, I sometimes forget to walk the dogs! The poor dogs shouldn't suffer because of my bad memory. It makes me wonder if I should quit my volunteer work."

Maintaining a certain amount of organization in your life will minimize both stress and confusion and allow your memory to work better. The real bonus of being organized is that with order, you'll find that you rely less and less on your memory. Take your medications at the same time every day, find a convenient place where you can *always* put your car keys, have special places for the things your regularly need, try making out your grocery list in the order that the items are found in your market, and in general, develop a routine that will encompass all those little things you tend to forget. Good habits can help make up for a less-than-perfect memory.

Eve's neighbor had known her for years and knew that Eve enjoyed her volunteering. He also was going through the same problem with his memory, but he'd discovered some tips that helped him. So he suggested that Eve do something very basic: make lists—for everything. That way, she could review her list periodically to make sure she wasn't forgetting something important. Plus, if she carried her daily list around with her, she'd always have paper on which to write reminders, shopping lists, and other important items.

It was so easy Eve couldn't believe she hadn't already tried it. Sure enough, she started making a daily to-do list—one personal, one for the animal shelter—and referred to it frequently. She started making fewer mistakes, and her self-confidence returned. If you call the animal shelter, she's still the enthusiastic voice on the other end.

Use Objects As Reminders

With their busy lives, it was easy for Barb and Steve to forget to walk the dogs when they returned home from work. They solved this problem by leaving the leashes in a prominent place when they went off to work in the morning. When they walked in the door at the end of the day, they couldn't miss the reminder.

Countless tricks like this will serve to jog your memory. If the weatherman says it's going to rain tomorrow, leave your umbrella hanging on the doorknob at night to remind yourself to take it with you in the morning. Try putting important correspondence on the keyboard of your computer, leave yourself a message on your own answering machine, or put a reminder in your shoe at night. The best places for reminders are where you can't miss them.

Leave Yourself Mental Notes

Rick leaves himself "mental notes" by "attaching" a mental reminder to a routine task. For instance, if Rick wants to

Maintaining a certain amount of organization will minimize stress and confusion, thus allowing your memory to function better.

remember the next morning to take the lunch he's packed and stored in the fridge, that evening he "attaches" a mental note to his briefcase. That is, he looks at the briefcase and tells himself that when he sees it in the morning, it will remind him to take his lunch. The next morning, when he starts to reach for his briefcase, a little mental reminder goes off: his lunch!

The trick is to associate the reminder with something you do every day. Associate your morning glass of orange juice with your daily medication, or tell yourself that when you open the

door to go to work tomorrow, you'll remember to bring along that something you promised to loan a co-worker. This works surprisingly well.

Using Developed Memory Techniques

People have been forgetting since humans first began to remember. Memory improvement techniques date back at least to the time of the ancient Greeks. Imagine how much more important memory must have been before everyone had paper and pencils and before literacy was common. In an oral tradition, our memories actually defined who we were. The stories shared over the generations were our history, and our guide to the present.

While many of the following techniques are designed for memorizing large numbers of items, they can work just as well for memorizing a handful of things. Play with each and see how well your mind adapts and how much each method helps you. These methods all require practice.

Visualization

This system has great potential and is marvelously easy. Simply associating things with images in your mind can be an amazing aid. Take the following list and match each set of items with an image:

frog	flag
shoe	ball
cat	bowl
flower	horse

Now close your eyes, visualize the images you have created and see if you are able to remember these items. Using absurd images can produce even better results: A cat in a bowl, a flower in a horse's ear, a empty shoe kicking a ball, and a frog waving a flag. You can use this technique to remember a shopping list by imagining an absurd "meal" of all the things on your list.

Storytelling

With this method, you simply create a story that includes what you want to remember. Try concocting a story with the elements of the above list.

Rhyming and Word Games

Creating rhymes and playing with words is a common method of remembering. You may not be aware of just how many of these memory aids you already use: "i before e except after c," "lock wise is clockwise," "30 days has September" . . . and so forth. Thousands of memory aids are created for every purpose from spelling ("The girl screamed **EEE!** as she passed the **CEMETERY**" to remember how to spell cemetery) to navigation ("Red on Right Returning"—to remember which way to turn when you come back from an errand in a strange city).

This system also works well with names. Having trouble remembering Bob Hartog? Have some fun and remember him as Bob Warthog. Ida Greenberg becomes I-ATE-A Greenbean. There's no end to this fun, as long as you remember not to call Bob, the new minister, Pastor Warthog.

Numbers work in much the same way. Take the locker combination 4 – 1 – 2. Remember that "For (4) one (1) to (2) get in the locker, one needs to know the combination." You can even make a game out of telephone numbers. Learn 283-5844 as "two [people] ate three eggs and five ate forty-four eggs." If you are mathematically inclined, you may find number relationships helpful. Play with numbers; thinking about them helps you to remember. It doesn't have to make sense. It only has to work for you.

For example, I remember the phone number 283-5844 like this: a phone number has two sections (2), eight digits total (8), and three digits in the first section (3). So there's the first part of the phone number (283). For me, the -5844 presents more of a problem until I realize that 8 is four twice (844) and 5 is one more than four, allowing me to remember -5844. Also you may have noticed that phone numbers punch out a pattern on a touch tone phone. Paying attention to this pattern can help you remember a phone number.

John's birthday is remembered by all his friends: December 3, 1945: 12/3/45 (1-2-3-4-5). Besides being helpful, such games can be entertaining and mentally stimulating.

Chunking

This is a simple way to remember numbers, and you've likely already used it. Chunking means remembering a large number by breaking it into smaller, more manageable groups. The number 382653086 would, for example, be more easily recalled as 382-653-086. Most people chunk best in groups of three; others manage larger clusters.

A variation of chunking would be to remember the number as $3,826,530.86. Here it's reduced to more manageable clusters and associated as a dollar amount, something even more easy to recall for some.

The Loci Method

The oldest system of memory improvement, the loci method, is based on the assumption that people can best remember familiar locations. It's an easy method to use and is especially effective if you have a vivid imagination. Here's how it works:

Pick a place that is very familiar to you. Most people find that their home works best. Mentally select a number of locations throughout it in the sequence that you would come to them. Now take the list of items you visualized earlier in this chapter (FROG, FLAG, SHOE, BALL, CAT, BOWL, FLOWER, and HORSE) and, in that order, imagine each one at the various locations you have chosen in your home. Don't just *think* about each one there but instead, use your imagination and *visualize* an image. Make each image more memorable by making it as absurd as you can. For example, imagine the frog selling flags door to door or the horse arranging flowers in the kitchen. Make a real effort to visualize, to really *see,* each image in your mind's eye.

Now simply take the trip around your home, and every time you come to one of your landmarks, you should be able to visualize the items from the list.

You will use these same locations each time you are memorizing a new list of items. The loci method was developed in Greece and was used by orators to remember their speeches. It is the source of the expression "In the first place."

First Letter Cueing.   The most common form of first letter cueing is the *acronym*. To create an acronym, simply take a list of things you're trying to remember and use the first letter of each to create a word. These shortcuts are everywhere in our world: MADD (Mothers Against Drunk Drivers), RAM (Random Access Memory), and NOW (National Organization of Women). It's easy to see how well these devices work. Some acronyms have actually become so commonly used that they have become words, for example NATO and scuba (which stands for self-contained underwater breathing apparatus). The trick with this method is to make up your own acronyms. Take the following shopping list and see what you can come up with:

grapes	raspberries
apples	soda
peas	

The other form of first letter cueing is called *acrostics*, and it means creating a sentence out of the first letters of a list of things. Generations of medical students have memorized anatomy with nonsense acrostics such as "On old Olympus terrace tops, a Finn and German viewed a hop." The first letters of each word of this phrase refers to the human cranial nerves. Using such devices has proven to be of great help to college students.

Try making an acrostic out of the above shopping list to see how this method works for you. If you find it easy, try making an acrostic from this list:

frog	flag
shoe	bird
book	

Repetition

Some memory is a learned skill. Repetition is part of practicing that skill. No matter how clever I may be in coming up with a way to remember a number or a list of words, I have to take advantage of repetition in order to get it into long-term memory. There is a natural rhythm to doing this. At first, the phrase or number naturally comes to mind a few minutes or an hour after learning it. This is a cue to repeat it and to take the time to go over it once or twice to make sure that I still remember it. Often, this is where you will discover that what you are remembering has begun to slip. At that point, make sure you get it right—and then forget about it. When it comes to mind again, and it will, quickly go over it. After a day or so, you may not think about it for a day or so more. When it does come to mind, take the trouble to repeat it and make sure it is correct. Within a week or two, you will find that it is well committed to memory.

Other Memory Techniques

There are many other memory techniques you can use to help you remember details. Among them are pegging, link systems, and the PQRST method. These systems all require considerably more learning and practice and seem better suited for academic purposes than for improving everyday memory. If you are interested in learning about them, libraries and bookstores have shelves of books on these subjects.

Fun and Games to Improve Your Memory

In one important respect, the mind *is* just like a muscle: you use it or you lose it. To keep your mind working well, there's no substitute for keeping it active. Play games with yourself and others to keep your thought processes going and growing. Here are some suggestions:

In one important respect, the mind *is* just like a muscle: *it's use it or lose it.*

- Play crosswords and word games.
- Go to the market with your shopping list and then don't look at it until you think you have everything on it.
- Play thinking games such as Scrabble and Trivial Pursuit or card games such as bridge.
- Try to memorize your bank account number. Don't forget to use chunking. After you've done it, move on to credit card numbers.
- From memory, try writing down all the phone numbers that you know (and who they belong to).
- Go through the year month by month and see how many birthdays you are able to recall.
- Get a computer and learn to use it for your finances or some other project.
- Play along with TV game shows that demand memory, such as *Jeopardy.*
- Read, take adult education courses, and keep your curiosity alive.

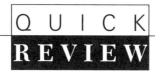

- Some basic steps to take to improve your memory are:
  1. Make a commitment to improve your memory.
  2. Have a positive attitude.
  3. Reduce stress.
  4. Focus on what you need to remember.
  5. Repeat the things you need to remember.
  6. Give understanding and meaning to what you are trying to remember.
  7. Talk to yourself out loud.
- Useful ways to help your memory are to make lists, get organized, give yourself visual reminders, use repetition, and make mental notes.
- Many specially developed memory techniques can help you remember details. These include visualization, storytelling, number chunking, the loci method, and first letter cueing.

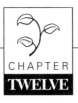

Putting It All Together

For your easy reference, this chapter contains a brief summary of the key practical information contained in this book. Please refer to earlier chapters for more comprehensive information, including a detailed discussion of safety issues.

The ginkgo tree is a unique and ancient species of tree. It has a long history in China of being used to treat a variety of conditions. In Europe, ginkgo has been an accepted medical treatment since at least the late 1980s. In Germany, it is a commonly prescribed drug used primarily to treat memory loss and mental decline.

Strong evidence tells us that ginkgo can protect memory and mental function in people with severe memory impairment, such as occurs in Alzheimer's disease. We don't know whether it can help the ordinary memory loss that occurs in all of us after 40, although there are logical reasons to think it might.

The typical dosage of ginkgo is 120 mg per day of an extract standardized to contain 24% flavonol glycosides and 6% terpene lactones. Ginkgo can take about 4 to 6 weeks to produce full benefits.

Extensive evidence indicates that ginkgo is a safe treatment when used correctly. However, there are a few concerns related to ginkgo's blood-thinning properties. People with a tendency toward bleeding should consult their doctor before taking ginkgo, and it should not be used just prior to or following surgery or labor and delivery. Also, if taking a blood-thinning medication such as warfarin (Coumadin), heparin, pentoxifylline (Trental), or aspirin, do not use ginkgo without first consulting your physician. It is conceivable that ginkgo could interact with mildly blood-thinning natural substances, such as garlic, phosphatidylserine (PS), and high dose vitamin E.

Ginkgo is also used for other conditions besides declining mental function, including intermittent claudication, PMS, impotence, some forms of tinnitus, one type of macular degeneration, and depression. Further, ginkgo may also act as an antidote against the sexual side effects caused by certain antidepressant drugs (impotence in men and inability to achieve orgasm in women) and help prevent and treat strokes and heart attacks. However, further research is necessary to firmly establish its value in treating any of these conditions.

Other Natural Treatments for Memory Loss

Besides ginkgo, there are other natural treatments that may help memory and mental function. Evidence strongly suggests that phosphytidylserine (PS) is an effective treatment for severe age-related memory loss, such as occurs with Alzheimer's disease. As with ginkgo, it may be helpful for ordinary age-related memory loss too, but this hasn't been proven.

The suggested dosage of PS is 100 mg 2 or 3 times a day. Once you experience good results using PS, you may find a lower dose of 100 mg daily to be sufficient.

PS is generally regarded as safe. However, as with ginkgo, if you are taking any blood-thinning or anti-coagulant herbs, supplements, or medications, consult with your physician before you take PS.

The natural substance L-acetylcarnitine may also be mildly helpful, taken at a dose of 500 mg to 1,000 mg 3 times a day. It appears to be very safe when taken at this dose.

Huperzine A and vinpocetine are "dietary supplements" that also appear to improve mental function, but they are really more like drugs than herbs. The herb ginseng may improve some aspects of thinking ability but does not appear to improve memory.

Conventional Treatments for Memory Loss

No prescription medications are available to treat ordinary age-related memory loss, but the two medications tacrine (Cognex) and donepezil (Aricept) have been approved for Alzheimer's disease. These medications don't reverse or prevent the disease, but they can improve mental functioning in about 30% of people with Alzheimer's disease.

Nonsteroidal anti-inflammatory drugs (NSAIDs) may reduce symptoms of Alzheimer's disease and also possibly slow its progression. Regular use of NSAIDs has also been associated with a lower overall incidence of Alzheimer's disease. However, these medications offer significant risks, and they should not be taken on a daily basis except on the advice of a physician.

Antioxidant substances such as selegiline and vitamin E appear to help slow the progression of Alzheimer's disease. Weak evidence suggests that regular use of estrogen reduces the chance of developing Alzheimer's disease.

Finally, though memory loss affects us all eventually, there are time-honored tips and techniques, as well as specially developed memory techniques that can help you remember better.

Notes

Chapter One

1. US Botanical Market Update. Herbalgram No. 44: 40.

2. Mabberley DJ. The plant book: a portable dictionary of the higher plants. Cambridge: Cambridge University Press, 1987: 242.

3. Pang Z, et al. *Ginkgo biloba L.:* History, current status, and future prospects. *J Altern Complement Med* 2: 359–363, 1996.

4. Schmid W. Ginkgo thrives. *Nature* 386: 755, 1997.

5. Huxtable RJ. The pharmacology of extinction. *J Ethnopharmacol* 37: 1–11, 1992.

6. DeFeudis FV. Ginkgo biloba extract (egb761): pharmacological activities and clinical applications. Paris: Elsevier, 1991: 2.

7. Schulz V. et al. Rational phytotherapy. New York: Springer-Verlag, 1998: 38.

8. Bauer R, Zschocke S. Medizinische Anwendung von *Ginkgo biloba* L. *Z Phytother* 17: 275–283, 1996.

9. van Beek TA, et al. *Ginkgo* L. *Fitoterapia* 69: 195–244, 1998.

Chapter Three

1. Small GW, et al. Diagnosis and treatment of Alzheimer's disease and related disorders: consensus statement of the American Association for Geriatric Psychiatry, the Alzheimer's Association, and the American Geriatrics Society. *JAMA* 278: 1363–1371, 1997.

2. Small GW, et al, 1997.

3. Hsiao KK. From prion diseases to Alzheimer's disease. *J Neural Transm Suppl* 49: 135–144, 1997.

4. Martyn CN, et al. Geographical relation between Alzheimer's disease and aluminum in drinking water. *Lancet* 8629: 59–62, 1989.

5. Bush AI, et al. Rapid induction of Alzheimer's A Beta amyloid formation by zinc. *Science* 265: 1464 –1467, 1994.

6. Knapp MJ, et al. A 30-week randomized controlled trial of high-dose tacrine in patients with Alzheimer's disease. The Tacrine Study Group. *JAMA* 271: 985–991, 1994.

Chapter Four

1. Youngjohn JR, et al. First-last names and the grocery list selective reminding test: two computerized measures of everyday verbal learning. *Arch Clin Neuropsychol* 6: 287–300, 1991.

2. Schulz V, et al. Rational phytotherapy. New York: Springer-Verlag, 1998: 246.

3. Le Bars PL, et al. A placebo-controlled, double-blind, randomized trial of an extract of Ginkgo for dementia. *JAMA* 278: 1327–1332, 1997.

4. Kleijnen J and Knipschild P. Ginkgo for cerebral insufficiency. *Br J Clin Pharmacol* 34: 352–358, 1992.

5. Hofferberth B. The efficacy of EGb 761 in patients with senile dementia of the Alzheimer type, a double-blind, placebo-controlled study on different levels of investigation. *Human Psychopharm* 9: 215–222, 1994.

6. Kanowski S, et al. Proof of efficacy of the *Ginkgo biloba* special extract EGb 761 in outpatients suffering from mild to moderate primary degenerative dementia of the Alzheimer type or multi-infarct dementia. *Pharmacopsychiatry* 29: 47–56, 1996.

7. Soholm B. Clinical improvement of memory and other cognitive functions by Ginkgo—review of relevant literature. *Adv Ther* 15: 54–65, 1998.

8. Schmidt U, et al. Einfluß eines *Ginkgo-biloba*-Spezialextraktes auf die Befindlichkeit bei zerebraler Insuffizienz (Effect of a *Ginkgo* special extract on the condition of patients with cerebral insufficiency). *Munch Med Wochenschr* 133(Suppl. 1): S15–S18, 1991.

9. Brüchert E, et al. Wirksamkeit von LI 1370 bei älteren Patienten mit Hirnleistungsschwäche. Multizentrische Doppelblind-studie des Fachverbandes Deutscher Allgemeinärzte (Effectiveness of LI 1370 in elderly patients with impaired cerebral function. Multicenter, double-blind study by the German Association of General Practitioners). *Münchener Medizinische Wochenschrift* 133(Suppl. 1): S9–S14, 1991.

10. Meyer B. Étude multicentrique randomisée à double insu face au placebo du traitement des acouphènes par l'extrait de Ginkgo (A multicenter, randomized, double-blind drug versus placebo study of *Ginkgo* extract in the treatment of tinnitus). *Presse Med* 15: 1562–1564, 1986.

11. Taillandier J, et al. Traitement des troubles du vieillissement cérébral par l'extrait de Ginkgo (*Ginkgo* extract in the treatment of cerebral disorders due to aging). *Presse Med* 15: 1583–1587, 1986.

12. Haguenauer JP, et al. Traitement des troubles de l'équilibre par l'extrait de Ginkgo. Etude multicentrique à double insu face as placebo (Treatment of disturbances of equilibrium with *Ginkgo* extract. A multicenter, double-blind, drug *versus* placebo study). *Presse Med* 15: 1569–1572, 1986.

13. Vorberg G, Schenk N, Schmidt U. Wirksamkeit eines neuen *Ginkgo-biloba*-Extracktes bei 100 Patient en mit zerebraler Insuffizienz (Effectiveness of a new *Ginkgo* extract in 100 patients with cerebral insufficiency). *Herz* 9: 936–941, 1989.

14. Eckmann F. Hirnleistungsstörungen-Behandlung mit *Ginkgo* Extrakt (Cerebral function disturbances—treatment with *Ginkgo* extract. Time of onset of action in a double-blind study with 60 inpatients). *Fortschr Med* 108: 557–560, 1990.

15. Wesnes K, et al. A double-blind placebo-controlled trial of Tanakan in the treatment of idiopathic cognitive impairment in the elderly. *Hum Psychopharmacol* 2: 159–169, 1987.

16. Koltringer P, et al. Hemorheologic effects and microcirculatory modifications following intravenous administration of ginkgo extract EGb 761. *Clin Hemorheol* 15: 649–656, 1995.

17. Erdincler DS, et al. The effect of ginkgo glycoside on the blood viscosity and erythrocyte deformability. *Clin Hemorheol* 16: 271–276, 1996.

18. Dumont E, et al. UV-C irradiation-induced peroxidative degradation of microsomal fatty acids and proteins: protec-

tion by an extract of ginkgo (EGb 761). *Free Radic Biol Med* 13: 197–203, 1992.

19. Dumont E, et al. Protection of polyunsaturated fatty acids against iron-dependent lipid peroxidation by a ginkgo extract (EGb 761). *Methods Find Exp Clin Pharmacol* 17: 83–88, 1995.

20. Barth SA, et al. Influences of Ginkgo on cyclosporin A induced lipid peroxidation in human liver microsomes in comparison to vitamin E, glutathione and N-acetylcysteine. *Biochem Pharmacol* 41: 1521–1526, 1991.

21. Kose K and Dogan P. Lipoperoxidation induced by hydrogen peroxide in human erythrocyte membranes. 1. Protective effect of ginkgo extract (EGb 761). *J Int Med Res* 23: 1–8, 1995.

22. Kose K and Dogan P. Lipoperoxidation induced by hydrogen peroxide in human erythrocyte membranes. 2. Comparison of the antioxidant effect of ginkgo extract (EGb 761) with those of water-soluble and lipid-soluble antioxidants. *J Int Med Res* 23: 9–18, 1995.

23. Kose K, et al. In vitro antioxidant effect of ginkgo extract (EGb 761) on lipoperoxidation induced by hydrogen peroxide in erythrocytes of Behcet's patients. *Jpn J Pharmacol* 75: 253–258, 1997.

24. Rong Y, et al. Ginkgo attenuates oxidative stress in macrophages and endothelial cells. *Free Radic Biol Med* 20: 121–127, 1996.

25. Oyama Y, et al. Ginkgo extract protects brain neurons against oxidative stress induced by hydrogen peroxide. *Brain Res* 712: 349–352, 1996.

26. Maitra I, et al. Peroxyl radical scavenging activity of ginkgo extract EGb 761. *Biochem Pharmacol* 49: 1649–1655, 1995.

27. Ramassamy C, et al. Ginkgo extract EGb 761 or trolox C prevent the ascorbic acid/Fe2+ induced decrease in synaptosomal membrane fluidity. *Free Radic Res Commun* 19: 341–350, 1993.

28. Yan LJ, et al. Ginkgo extract (EGb 761) protects human low density lipoproteins against oxidative modification mediated by copper. *Biochem Biophys Res Commun* 212: 360–366, 1995.

29. Schulz V, et al. 1998.

30. Spinnewyn B, et al. Involvement of platelet-activating factor (PAF) in cerebral post-ischemic phase in Mongolian gerbils. *Prostaglandins* 34: 337–349, 1987.

31. Hindmarch I. Activité de l'extrait de ginkgo sur la mémoire à court terme (Activity of ginkgo extract on short term memory). *Presse Med* 15: 1592–1594, 1986.

32. Subhan Z and Hindmarch I. The psychopharmacological effects of ginkgo extract in normal healthy volunteers. *Int J Clin Pharmacol Res* 4: 89–93, 1984.

Chapter Five

1. Sticher O. Quality of *Ginkgo* Preparations. *Planta Med* 59: 2–11, 1993.

2. DeFeudis FV. Ginkgo biloba Extract (EGb761): Pharmacological Activities and Clinical Applications. Paris: Elsevier, 12, 1991.

3. Bonati A, 1991. How and why should we standardize phytopharmaceutical drugs for clinical validation? *Ethnopharmacol* 32: 195–197, 1991.

Chapter Six

1. Kleijnen J and Knipschild P. Ginkgo biloba for cerebral insufficiency. *Br J Clin Pharmacol* 34: 352–358, 1992.

2. DeFeudis FV. Ginkgo biloba Extract (EGb 761): Pharmacological Activities and Clinical Applications. Paris: Elsevier, 143–146, 1991.

3. Schulz V, et al. Rational phytotherapy. New York: Springer-Verlag, 1998: 48.

4. DeFeudis FV. 1991.

5. Rowin J and Lewis SL. Spontaneous bilateral subdural hematomas associated with chronic *Ginkgo biloba* ingestion. *Neurology* 46: 1775–1776, 1996.

6. Gilbert GJ. *Ginkgo biloba* (letter). *Neurology* 48: 1137, 1997.

7. Odawara M, et al. *Ginkgo biloba* (letter). *Neurology* 48: 789–790, 1997.

8. Rosenblatt M and Mindel J. Spontaneous hyphema associated with ingestion of *Ginkgo biloba* extract. *N Engl J Med* 336: 1108, 1997.

9. DeFeudis FV. 1991.

Chapter Seven

1. Peters H, et al. Demonstration of the efficacy of *Ginkgo biloba* special extract EGb 761 on intermittent claudication—a placebo-controlled, double-blind multicenter trial. *Vasa* 27: 106–110, 1998.

2. Blume J, et al. Placebo-controlled double-blind study of the effectiveness of *Ginkgo biloba* special extract EGb 761 in trained patients with intermittent claudication (in German). *Vasa* 25: 265–274, 1996.

3. Kleijnen J and Knipschild P. Ginkgo biloba for cerebral insufficiency. *Br J Clin Pharmacol* 34: 352–358, 1992.

4. Tamborini A, et al. Value of standardized *Ginkgo biloba* extract (Egb761) in the management of congestive symptoms of premenstrual syndrome. *Rev Fr Gynecol Obstet* 88: 447–457, 1993.

5. Lebuisson DA, et al. Treatment of senile macular degeneration with *Ginkgo Biloba* extract. A preliminary double-blind study versus placebo. *Rökan (Ginkgo biloba).* In *Recent Results in Pharmacology and Clinic.* Fünfgeld EW, ed. New York: Springer-Verlag, 1988: 231–236.

6. Doly M, et al. Oxidative stress in diabetic retina. *EXS* 62: 299–307, 1992.

7. Szabo ME, et al. Direct measurement of free radicals in ischemic/reperfused diabetic rat retina. *Clin Neurosci* 4: 240–245, 1997.

8. Meyer B. Multicenter randomized double-blind drug vs. placebo study of the treatment of tinnitus with *Ginkgo biloba* extract (in French). *Presse Med* 15: 1562–1564, 1986.

9. Holgers KM, et al. *Ginkgo biloba* extract for the treatment of tinnitus. *Audiology* 33: 85–92, 1994.

10. Coles RRA. Trial of an extract of *Ginkgo biloba* (EGB) for tinnitus and hearing loss. *Clin Otolaryngol* 13: 501–504, 1988.

11. Sohn M and Sikora R. *Ginkgo biloba* extract in the therapy of erectile dysfunction. *J Sex Educ Ther* 17: 53–61, 1991.

12. Cohen AJ and Bartlik B. *Ginkgo biloba* for antidepressant-induced sexual dysfunction. *J Sex Marital Ther* 24: 139–143, 1988.

13. Schubert H, et al. Depressive episode primarily unresponsive to therapy in elderly patients: Efficacy of *Ginkgo biloba* extract (EGb 761) in combination with antidepressants. *Geriatr Forsch* 3: 45–53, 1993.

14. Seif-El-Nasr M and El-Fattah AA. Lipid peroxide, phospholipids, glutathione levels and superoxide dismutase activity in rat brain after ischaemia: effect of ginkgo extract. *Pharmacol Res* 32: 273–278, 1995.

15. Koc RK, et al. Lipid peroxidation in experimental spinal cord injury. Comparison of treatment with ginkgo, TRH and methylprednisolone. *Res Exp Med (Berl)* 195: 117–123, 1995.

16. Shen JG and Zhou DY. Efficiency of Ginkgo extract (EGb 761) in antioxidant protection against myocardial ischemia and reperfusion injury. *Biochem Mol Biol Int* 35: 125–134, 1995.

17. Haramaki N, et al. Effects of natural antioxidant ginkgo extract (EGB 761) on myocardial ischemia-reperfusion injury. *Free Radic Biol Med* 16: 789–794, 1994.

18. Pietri S, et al. Cardioprotective and anti-oxidant effects of the terpene constituents of Ginkgo extract (EGb 761). *J Mol Cell Cardiol* 29: 733–742, 1997.

19. Oyama Y, et al. Myricetin and quercetin, the flavonoid constituents of Ginkgo extract, greatly reduce oxidative metabolism in both resting and $Ca(2+)$-loaded brain neurons. *Brain Res* 635: 125–129, 1994.

20. Brailowsky S, et al. Acceleration of functional recovery from motor cortex ablation by Ginkgo extracts in rats. *Restorative Neurol Neurosci* 8: 163–167, 1995.

Chapter Eight

1. Cenacchi T, et al. Cognitive decline in the elderly: a double-blind, placebo-controlled multicenter study on efficacy of phosphatidylserine administration. *Aging (Milano)* 5: 123–133, 1993.

2. Amaducci L. Phosphatidylserine in the treatment of Alzheimer's disease: results of a multicenter study. *Psychopharmacol Bull* 24: 130–134, 1988.

3. Crook T, et al. Effects of phosphatidylserine in Alzheimer's disease. *Psychopharmacol Bull* 28: 61–66, 1992.

4. Crook T, et al. Effects of phosphatidylserine in age-associated memory impairment. *Neurology* 41: 644–649, 1991.

5. Delwaide PJ, et al. Double-blind randomized controlled study of phosphatidylserine in senile demented patients. *Acta Neurol Scand* 73: 136–140, 1986.

6. Nerozzi D, et al. Phosphatidylserine and memory disorders in the aged (in Italian). *Clin Ther* 120: 399–404, 1987.

7. Palmieri G, et al. Double-blind controlled trial of phosphatidylserine in subjects with senile mental deterioration. *Clin Trials J* 24: 73–83, 1987.

8. Villardita C, et al. Multicentre clinical trial of brain phosphatidylserine in elderly subjects with mental deterioration. *Clin Trials J* 24: 84–93, 1987.

9. Engel RR, et al. Double-blind crossover study of phosphatidylserine vs. placebo in subjects with early cognitive deterioration of the Alzheimer type. *Eur Neuropsychopharmacol* 2: 149–155, 1992.

10. Palatini P, et al. Pharmacokinetic characterization of phosphatidylserine liposomes in the rat. *Br J Pharmacol* 102: 345–350, 1991.

11. Martin SJ, et al. Early redistribution of plasma membrane phosphatidylserine is a general feature of apoptosis regardless of the initiating stimulus: inhibition by overexpression of Bcl-2 and Abl. *J Exp Med* 182: 1545–1556, 1995.

12. Martin SJ, et al. Phosphatidylserine externalization during CD95-induced apoptosis of cells and cytoplasts requires ICE/CED-3 protease activity. *J Biol Chem* 271: 28753–28756, 1996.

13. Casamenti F, et al. Phosphatidylserine reverses the age-dependent decrease in cortical acetylcholine release: a microdialysis study. *Eur J Pharmacol* 194: 11–16, 1991.

14. Casamenti F, et al. Effect of phosphatidylserine on acetyl-choline output from the cerebral cortex of the rat. *J Neurochem* 32: 529–533, 1979.

15. van den Besselaar AM. Phosphatidylethanolamine and phosphatidylserine synergistically promote heparin's anticoagulant effect. *Blood Coagul Fibrinolysis* 6: 239–244, 1995.

Chapter Nine

1. Carta A, et al. Acetyl-L-carnitine and Alzheimer's disease: pharmacological considerations beyond the cholinergic sphere. *Ann N Y Acad Sci* 695: 324–326, 1993.

2. Carta A and Calvani M. Acetyl-L-carnitine: a drug able to slow the progress of Alzheimer's disease? *Ann N Y Acad Sci* 640: 228–232, 1991.

3. Parnetti L, et al. Pharmacokinetics of IV and oral acetyl-L-carnitine in a multiple dose regimen in patients with senile dementia of Alzheimer type. *Eur J Clin Pharmacol* 42: 89–93, 1992.

4. Calvani M, et al. Action of acetyl-L-carnitine in neurodegeneration and Alzheimer's disease. *Ann N Y Acad Sci* 663: 483–486, 1992.

5. Sano M, et al. Double-blind parallel design pilot study of acetyl levocarnitine in patients with Alzheimer's disease. *Arch Neurol* 49: 1137–1141, 1992.

6. Campi N, et al. Selegiline versus L-acetylcarnitine in the treatment of Alzheimer-type dementia. *Clin Ther* 12: 306–314, 1990.

7. Garzya G, et al. Evaluation of the effects of L-acetylcarnitine on senile patients suffering from depression. *Drugs Exp Clin Res* 16: 101–106, 1990.

8. Vecchi GP, et al. Methodology of a controlled clinical study for cerebral aging evaluation. *Int J Clin Pharmacol Res* 10: 145–152, 1990.

9. Passeri M, et al. Acetyl-L-carnitine in the treatment of mildly demented elderly patients. *Int J Clin Pharmacol Res* 10: 75–79, 1990.

10. Spagnoli A, et al. Long-term acetyl-L-carnitine treatment in Alzheimer's disease. *Neurology* 41: 1726–1732, 1991.

11. Rai G, et al. Double-blind, placebo controlled study of acetyl-l-carnitine in patients with Alzheimer's dementia. *Curr Med Res Opin* 11: 638–467, 1990.

12. Bonavita E. Study of the efficacy and tolerability of L-acetylcarnitine therapy in the senile brain. *Int J Clin Pharmacol Ther Toxicol* 24: 511–516, 1986.

13. Bella R, et al. Effect of acetyl-L-carnitine on geriatric patients suffering from dysthymic disorders. *Int J Clin Pharmacol Res* 10: 355–360, 1990.

14. Spagnoli, et al. 1991.

15. Calvani M, et al, 1992.

16. Salvioli G and Neri M. L-acetylcarnitine treatment of mental decline in the elderly. *Drugs Exp Clin Res* 20: 169–176, 1994.

17. Cipolli C, et al. Effects of L-acetylcarnitine on mental deterioration in the aged: Initial results. *Clin Ther* 132: 479–510, 1990.

18. Thal LJ, et al. A 1-year multicenter placebo-controlled study of acetyl-L-carnitine in patients with Alzheimer's disease. *Neurology* 47: 705–711, 1996.

19. Zhang RW, et al. Drug evaluation of huperzine A in the treatment of senile memory disorders (in Chinese). *Chung Kuo Yao Li Hsueh Pao* 12: 250–252, 1991.

20. Raves ML, et al. Structure of acetylcholinesterase complexed with the nootropic alkaloid, (-)-huperzine A. *Nat Struct Biol* 4: 57–63, 1997.

21. Ashani Y, et al. Mechanism of inhibition of cholinesterases by huperzine A. *Biochem Biophys Res Commun* 184: 719–726, 1992.

22. Pang YP and Kozikowski AP. Prediction of the binding sites of huperzine A in acetylcholinesterase by docking studies. *J Comput Aided Mol Des* 8: 669–681, 1994.

23. Cheng DH and Tang XC. Comparative studies of huperzine A, E2020, and tacrine on behavior and cholinesterase activities. *Pharmacol Biochem Behav* 60: 377–386, 1998.

24. Cheng DH et al. Huperzine A, a novel promising acetylcholinesterase inhibitor. *Neuroreport* 8: 97–101, 1996.

25. Xiong ZQ and Tang XC. Effect of huperzine A, a novel acetylcholinesterase inhibitor, on radial maze performance in rats. *Pharmacol Biochem Behav* 51: 415–419, 1995.

26. Zhi QX, et al. Huperzine A ameliorates the spatial working memory impairments induced by AF64A. *Neuroreport* 6: 2221–2224, 1995.

27. Zhu XD and Giacobini E. Second generation cholinesterase inhibitors: effect of (L)-huperzine-A on cortical biogenic amines. *J Neurosci Res* 41: 828–835, 1995.

28. Zhang GB, et al. Facilitation of cholinergic transmission by huperzine A in toad paravertebral ganglia in vitro (in Chinese). *Chung Kuo Yao Li Hsueh Pao* 15: 158–161, 1994.

29. Laganiere S, et al. Acute and chronic studies with the anti-cholinesterase Huperzine A: effect on central nervous system cholinergic parameters. *Neuropharmacology* 30: 763–768, 1991.

30. Tang XC, et al. Effect of huperzine A, a new cholinesterase inhibitor, on the central cholinergic system of the rat. *J Neurosci Res* 24: 276–285, 1989.

31. Tang XC, et al. Effects of huperzine A on learning and the retrieval process of discrimination performance in rats (in Chinese). *Chung Kuo Yao Li Hsueh Pao* 7: 507–511, 1986.

32. Guan LC, et al. Effects of huperzine A on electroencephalography power spectrum in rabbits (in Chinese). *Chung Kuo Yao Li Hsueh Pao* 10: 496–500, 1989.

33. Lu WH, et al. Improving effect of huperzine A on discrimination performance in aged rats and adult rats with experimental cognitive impairment (in Chinese). *Chung Kuo Yao Li Hsueh Pao* 9: 11–15, 1988.

34. Wang YE, et al. Pharmacokinetics of huperzine A in rats and mice (in Chinese). *Chung Kuo Yao Li Hsueh Pao* 9: 193–196, 1988.

35. Wang YE, et al. Anti-cholinesterase activity of huperzine A (in Chinese). *Chung Kuo Yao Li Hsueh Pao* 7: 110–113, 1986.

36. Zhu XD and Tang XC. Improvement of impaired memory in mice by huperzine A and huperzine B (in Chinese). *Chung Kuo Yao Li Hsueh Pao* 9: 492–497, 1988.

37. Zhu XD and Tang XC. Facilitatory effects of huperzine A and B on learning and memory of spatial discrimination in mice (in Chinese). *Yao Hsueh Hsueh Pao* 22: 812–817, 1987.

38. Yan XF, et al. Effects of huperzine A and B on skeletal muscle and the electroencephalogram (in Chinese). *Chung Kuo Yao Li Hsueh Pao* 8: 117–123, 1987.

39. Xu SS, et al. Efficacy of tablet huperzine-A on memory, cognition, and behavior in Alzheimer's disease. *Chung Kuo Yao Li Hsueh Pao* 16: 391–395, 1995.

40. Bruneton J. Pharmacognosy, Phytochemistry, Medicinal Plants. Paris: Lavoisier Publishing, 838–840, 844, 1995.

41. Kiss B, et al. Mechanism of action of vinpocetine. *Acta Pharm Hung* 66(5): 213–14, 1996.

42. Balestreri R, et al. A double-blind placebo controlled evaluation of the safety and efficacy of vinpocetine in the treatment of patients with chronic vascular senile cerebral dysfunction. *J Am Geriatr Soc* 35: 425–430, 1987.

43. Hindmarch I, Fuchs HH, and Erzigkeit. Efficacy and tolerance of vinpocetine in ambulant patients suffering from mild to moderate organic psychosyndromes. *Int Clin Psychopharmacol* 6: 31–43, 1991.

44. Thal LJ, et al. The safety and lack of efficacy of vinpocetine in Alzheimer's disease. *J Am Geriatr Soc* 37: 515–520, 1989.

45. Lohmann A, et al. Bioavailability of vinpocetine and interference of the time of application with food intake. *Arzneimittelforschung* 42: 914–917, 1992.

46. Hitzenberger G, et al. Influence of vinpocetine on warfarin-induced inhibition of coagulation. *Int J Clin Pharmacol Ther Toxicol* 28: 323–328, 1990.

47. Sorenson H, et al. A double-masked study of the effects of ginseng on cognitive functions. *Curr Ther Res Clin Exp* 57(12): 959–68, 1996.

Chapter Ten

1. Giacobini E. Invited review: Cholinesterase inhibitors for Alzheimer's disease therapy: from tacrine to future applications. *Neurochem Int* 32: 413–419, 1998.

2. Giacobini E, 1998.

3. Rogers J, et al. Clinical trial of indomethacin in Alzheimer's disease. *Neurology* 43: 1609–1611, 1993.

4. Rich JB, et al. Nonsteroidal anti-inflammatory drugs in Alzheimer's disease. *Neurology* 45: 51–55, 1995.

5. Breitner JC. Inflammatory processes and antiinflammatory drugs in Alzheimer's disease: a current appraisal. *Neurobiol Aging* 17: 789–794, 1996.

6. Sano M, et al. A controlled trial of selegiline, alpha-tocopherol, or both as treatment for Alzheimer's disease. The Alzheimer's Disease Cooperative Study. *N Engl J Med* 336: 1216–1222, 1997.

7. Baldereschi M, et al. Estrogen-replacement therapy and Alzheimer's disease in the Italian Longitudinal Study on Aging. *Neurology* 50: 996–1002, 1998.

8. Kawas C, et al. A prospective study of estrogen replacement therapy and the risk of developing Alzheimer's disease: the Baltimore Longitudinal Study of Aging. *Neurology* 48: 1517–1521, 1997.

9. Paganini-Hill A and Henderson VW. Estrogen replacement therapy and risk of Alzheimer disease. *Arch Intern Med* 156: 2213–2217, 1996.

10. Tang MX, et al. Effect of estrogen during menopause on risk and age at onset of Alzheimer's disease. *Lancet* 348: 429–432, 1996.

11. Birge SJ. The role of estrogen in the treatment of Alzheimer's disease. *Neurology* 48: S36–S41, 1997.

12. Haskell SG, et al. The effect of estrogen replacement therapy on cognitive function in women: a critical review of the literature. *J Clin Epidemiol* 50: 1249–1264, 1997.

13. Johnson SR. Menopause and hormone replacement therapy. *Med Clin North Am* 82: 297–320, 1998.

14. Smalheiser NR and Swanson DR. Linking estrogen to Alzheimer's disease: an informatics approach. *Neurology* 47: 809–810, 1996.

15. Schneider LS and Olin JT. Overview of clinical trials of hydergine in dementia. *Arch Neurol* 51: 787–798, 1994.

Index

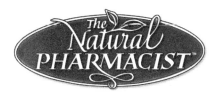

About the Author

Steven Dentali, Ph.D., is former president of Dentali Associates, which specialized in natural products consulting for industry and government. He has also worked in research and development and quality assurance positions in the herbal industry.

Dentali has served as a reviewer for the NIH office of Alternative Medicine and as an adviser to the FDA. He is currently an advisory board member of the American Botanical Council. He recently became senior director of botanical sciences for Rexall Sundown.

About the Series Editors

Steven Bratman, M.D., medical director of Prima Health, has many years of experience in the alternative medicine field. A graduate of the University of California at Davis, Medical School, he has also trained in herbology, nutrition, Chinese medicine, and other alternative therapies, and has worked closely with a wide variety of alternative practitioners. He is the author of *The Natural Pharmacist: Your Complete Guide to Herbs* (Prima), *The Natural Pharmacist: Your Complete Guide to Illnesses and Their Natural Remedies* (Prima), *The Natural Pharmacist Guide to St. John's Wort and Depression* (Prima), *The Alternative Medicine Ratings Guide* (Prima), and *The Alternative Medicine Sourcebook* (Lowell House).

David J. Kroll, Ph.D., is a professor of pharmacology and toxicology at the University of Colorado School of Pharmacy and a consultant for pharmacists, physicians, and alternative practitioners on the indications and cautions for herbal medicine use. A graduate of both the University of Florida and the Philadelphia College of Pharmacy and Science, Dr. Kroll has lectured widely and has published articles in a number of medical journals, abstracts, and newsletters.